6-Minute Sana-Facial-Exercises™ & Face-Care Program for Women

1st printing—September 1971
2nd printing—September 1971
3rd printing—April 1972
4th printing—May 1972
5th printing—June 1972
6th printing—September 1972

Manufactured in the United States of America

Trademarks pending in the U.S. Patent Office for Source Publishers, Inc.

Library of Congress Catalogue Card Number: 78-175096

ISBN: 0-87915-006-8

by Grace Jane Treber

Books by Grace Jane Treber

SANASESSION™ 4 Minute Effortless, Inches Off & Slimming Program for Men and Women

> A proven method to slim, trim inches from upper arms, spare tire, waist, stomach, upper legs, hips. Firms flabbiness. Shape up and be fit. No soreness afterwards. No straining. The author lost 40 lbs. in 2 months without dieting, 8″ from hips, 3″ from upper thighs. 3-Part program $10.00

6-Minute SANA-FACIAL-EXERCISES™ for Men

> Easy-to-do-and-remember face exercises—natural face lifting. Helps get rid of double chin, helps tighten sagging, firms $4.95

WHY KILL TO EAT™—500 gourmet recipes

> Appetizers, hors d'oeuvres, soups, salads, vegetables, desserts, omelettes, etc. Complete with special sections on cheeses, teas, coffees. Most of the recipes take under 20 minutes. All recipes tested—easy to do whether you've cooked before or not. 1 dish gourmet meals and 7 course epicurean delights. How to be supper hostess (and enjoy doing it) $3.95

SOURCE PUBLISHERS, INC., 239 EAST 52 STREET • NEW YORK, NEW YORK 10022, U.S.A. • TELEPHONE (212) 838-2333

Contents

Why the Face Ages

Four major processes account for the differences between an old and a young face:

1. The skeletal framework thins with age and requires less space.
2. The natural lines of expression and action of the face and neck deepen, and become more obvious.
3. The skin becomes lax and sags into folds and pouches.
4. Skin color-changes.

Squinting, laughing and frowning are not problems in the very young because a moist skin can't crease. The drying process which begins at adolescence clearly starts to age the skin.

Aging skin markedly loses fat and tissue fluid; there is a weakening of structure, and a corresponding loss of function of the sebaceous and sweat glands.

Skin elasticity also starts to disappear. This elasticity is due to elastic fibers in the Dermis and Subcutaneous layers of the skin. With age the total connective tissue becomes thin and inelastic, and the fatty tissue is absorbed which causes uneven folds (wrinkles).

Other Causes of Aging

The weather and its variances effect change: excessive heat, humidity or cold, excessively dry air—all take a toll. Even the indoor heating in your home dries the skin and drying causes wrinkles. Outdoors the air itself carries city soot, grime, and a broad selection of pollutants, all bringing about skin changes.

Too much sun is a prime factor in the drying and aging of skin. Neglect (the lack of proper cleansing and moisturizing), deep emotional stress, illness, medication, loss of sleep, improper diet, not taking a cold shower after a steam bath or sauna, not drying all water from the skin, a lack of proper health precautions can all cause facial aging.

Finally, habits of expression such as constant and prolonged frowning, raised eyebrows, etc., can impress lines where none should be.

How to Help Slow Aging

According to leading experts nothing will rid one permanently of the varied problems due to aging, but certain preventive measures can slow the process.

Cleansing—basis for all good skin care. Most people cleanse but don't do total cleansing.

Creaming—smooths and softens only; 20 minutes does maximum good.

Moisturizing—keeps skin from drying. Drying causes wrinkles. Use at all times even under make-up and at night.

Facial massage—relaxes, and in conjunction with cream or oil, softens.

Proper nutrition—promotes good cell reproduction and healthy cell growth. Helps give a naturally radiant, glowing complexion.

A few minutes each day with a face-care and exercise program incorporating the above will give big dividends and prove more valuable than an hour once a week.

All complexions, regardless of age, will benefit since the skin renews and replenishes itself with proper care.

Great faces don't just happen. Women with great beauty adhere to a regular daily beauty regime in order to achieve and maintain their lovely smooth complexions. The key to their success is knowing what they're doing, and applying intensive, knowledgeable, consistent care. We may not be able to stop aging, but we certainly can slow it down. Envision the glamorous movie-star grandmothers and let's waste no more time.

LET'S FIND OUT . . .!

Face-Care Program

What the Skin Is All About

The skin's primary function is protection: protection from injury to the more sensitive tissues within; from invasion by foreign organisms, as bacteria; from all injurious elements of the environment including the rays of the sun. It is a sense organ, supplied with nerves and nerve receptors, constantly reacting to the conditions that surround it. Thus it regulates body temperature through the controlled loss of heat. It also functions as a place of storage for certain materials. (The skin comprises $\frac{1}{12}$ of the total body mass, and represents a surface area of more than 3000 square inches on the average adult. About 20 percent of one's protein requirements are used to replace skin cells.)

Though your facial-skin surface may appear smooth, if you examined it under a magnifying glass, you'd see ridges, valleys, and patterns of skin texture. These reflect the total depth of the skin and its composition.

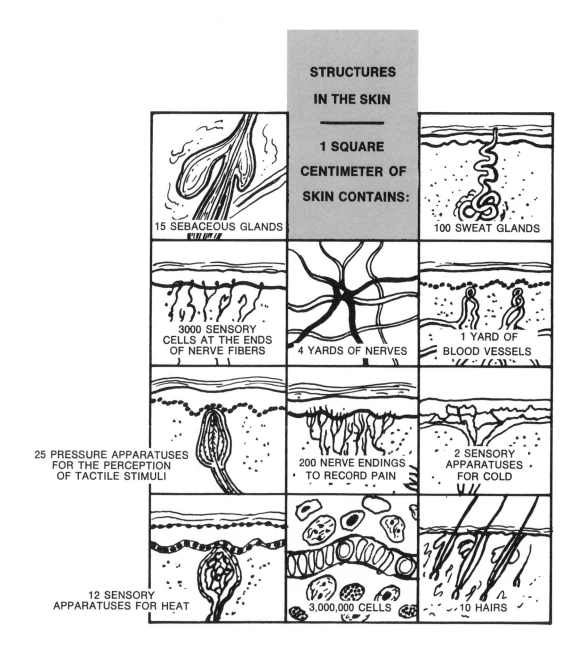

STRUCTURES

IN THE SKIN

———

1 SQUARE

CENTIMETER OF

SKIN CONTAINS:

15 SEBACEOUS GLANDS

100 SWEAT GLANDS

3000 SENSORY
CELLS AT THE ENDS
OF NERVE FIBERS

4 YARDS OF NERVES

1 YARD OF
BLOOD VESSELS

25 PRESSURE APPARATUSES
FOR THE PERCEPTION
OF TACTILE STIMULI

200 NERVE ENDINGS
TO RECORD PAIN

2 SENSORY
APPARATUSES
FOR COLD

12 SENSORY
APPARATUSES FOR HEAT

3,000,000 CELLS

10 HAIRS

Skin Composition

The skin is composed of three layers of tissue.

The Subcutaneous

The subcutaneous, or inner-most layer, is a fatty tissue that links the dermis (middle layer) with the tissues covering the muscles and bones. It acts as a springy smooth cushion and protects nerves, glands, and blood vessels.

The Dermis (Corium)

The dermis, or middle layer, varies in thickness. It contains nerves, nerve receptors, and hair follicles; its sweat glands, oil glands, and blood vessels bring nourishment to the upper skin cells. The dermis is composed of dense connective tissue which becomes more open in texture in its deeper parts where it merges with the subcutaneous layer. (The elasticity of the skin is due to the presence, in the dermis and subcutaneous layers, of numerous fine elastic fibers.) At the top of the dermis, millions of cone-shaped papillae mesh with the ridged underside of the epidermis (the visible skin tissue) to secure the layers of skin from slipping.

The Epidermis

The epidermis, or outer skin, is a tissue which is constantly being renewed. Its surface is a sheet of scales and dead skin cells. These flake or soak off when wet and are replaced by new cells from the underlying layers. The replacement is not a periodic event, but a continuous assembly-line process, with cells at each stage of production arranged in layers. Current research indicates that all the cells of the epidermis are replaced in man about once each month. It is a constant movement of cells through division, migration, differentiation—to death, and the apparent purpose of all this action is the healthy maintenance of an efficient barrier to protect the individual from his external environment. The foundation of the barrier is protein. The epidermis, or outer (facial) skin, differs in type from one individual to another.

Basic Facial-Skin Types

There are different basic facial-skin types—oily, dry, combination, sensitive, sensitive allergic. Your skin is susceptible to change from almost any influence inside or outside the body; adolescence, for example; pregnancy, menopause, age, nervous tension or emotional stress; nutrition and medication.

Since there is a continual process of cell replacement, and since the facial skin must "breathe" through its pores, you can understand how important a daily face-care program is, no matter what your skin type, and the most important part of this program is cleansing.

Regular cleansing is essential because it removes oil secretions (sebum), perspiration, dead skin, dirt, cosmetics, and bacteria.

There are different types of cleansers. whipped cleansing creams, cold creams, cleansing oils, and liquids, etc. Read the labels carefully and choose the one that suits your skin type best. You may have to experiment with several kinds before you find the one best for you. Never apply new make-up over old, always clean old make-up off face with cleanser.

Most authorities feel soap should be used at least once every 24 hours on the skin. Experiment with several mild complexion soaps until you find one best for your skin type. Use a mild complexion soap with a genuine natural-bristle complexion brush. If the correct kind of mild complexion soap is used, and thoroughly rinsed off (rinsing off *all* soap is vitally important), if water is neither too hot nor too cold, women with dry skin should have no problems using soap once a day. If irritation occurs, however, discontinue soap and use only cleanser. Authorities feel oily skin should be washed 3 to 6 times a day, whenever oiliness appears. Follow the skin-care program carefully and consistently for your skin type.

When choosing a complexion brush make sure the bristles are natural, and are the texture (softness) that you require for your skin. Rinse the brush thoroughly after use. Use brush only once a day. If

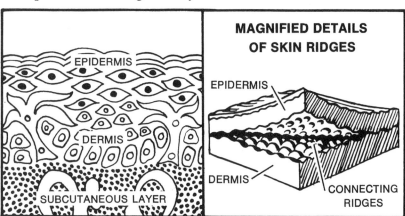

MAGNIFIED DETAILS
OF SKIN RIDGES

EPIDERMIS

DERMIS

SUBCUTANEOUS LAYER

EPIDERMIS

DERMIS

CONNECTING
RIDGES

you use soap more than once a day, use fingers to lather on for subsequent washings. Washcloths may gather bacteria, so washing with fingertips is suggested. However, if you would rather use a cloth, do. Just be sure it is always immaculately clean. Between using, rinse and wring it out well. Hang your washcloth where it will get plenty of air and light.

If you wish to use a mild skin freshener (dry skin), or a mild astringent (oily skin), do so after the rinsing and the splashes in the skin-care program. Then dry and apply moisturizer.

The frequency of application of moisturizer is very important. Moisturizer should be used at all times after every cleansing, under make-up and at night as moisturizer helps prevent drying and drying causes wrinkles. Make sure, however, you have a moisturizer and not a face cream. Moisturizer carefully chosen for your skin type does not make oily skin oilier, it just helps prevent drying for all skin types. Use often and liberally.

When choosing face creams, evaluate on an individual basis. Usually an all-purpose face cream for oily skin, a dry-skin face cream for a dry or combination skin. Many women with oily skin think cream will make their skin more oily. It won't, if chosen carefully for that skin type. Remember, creams only smooth and soften. That's all they can accomplish. Most authorities feel 20 minutes give maximum benefit as the skin can't absorb more than it does in that time.

Masks are excellent for oily skins. Read labels carefully and select according to your own skin type, and what you wish to accomplish.

Discontinue the use of any product that causes unusual redness or irritation.

One must exert extreme care with facial skin. Avoid extremes of any kind (hot or cold, ice or steam) directly on the face. In a steam bath or sauna always have cream on your neck and face. Do not use "anything" above your chin except your fingertips and use them with featherlike lightness. And remember: don't rub under the eyes, don't apply masks around the eye area. With the gentlest fingertips movement dot on moisturizers and creams, and treat the skin in this area most gently and carefully. Never scrub, rub, slap, or use any heavy stroking or pulling on your face. Don't use machines directly on the facial skin. Chin straps are a waste of time — accomplish nothing.

No matter what facial-skin type you are, the daily following of this down-to-earth program for your skin type will produce, within just a few weeks, a radiant and glowing complexion, a beautiful natural look. Wonders can be worked! And make-up then is up to you.

Techniques of Application

How to cleanse and tissue off

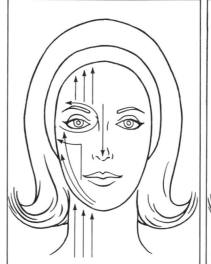

How to apply cream and moisturizer

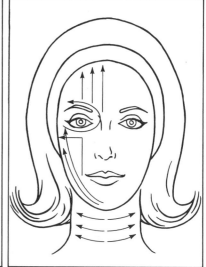

Know Your Skin Type

Dry Skin	Feels tight and drawn Has a fine textured look Peels, chaps, flakes easily
Oily Skin	Often coarse textured Oily especially around the chin, nose, and forehead
Combination Skin	Some parts oily, some parts dry, some parts normal
Sensitive Skin	Thin, transparent, often reacts unfavorably, "flares up," to certain ingredients in products that would not bother normal skin
Sensitive-Allergic Skin	See a dermatologist

Dry Skin-Care Program

Morning

ALWAYS WASH HANDS BEFORE TOUCHING FACE.

Cleanse neck and face with mild, non-drying complexion soap, use fingers to lather on, use a natural-bristle complexion brush gently.

Using fingers, rinse off thoroughly with lukewarm water.

Then splash neck and face 30 times with cool water.

Dry neck and face.

Apply dry-skin cream to neck and face.

Leave on. Take your morning shower or bath.

After this, tissue off cream gently.

Using fingers, rinse neck and face thoroughly with lukewarm water.

Then splash neck and face 30 times with cool water.

Dry neck and face.

Apply moisturizer liberally to neck and face.

Blot lightly with tissue.

You're now ready to apply make-up.

Evening

ALWAYS WASH HANDS BEFORE TOUCHING FACE.

Cleanse neck and face with whatever cleanser you prefer. Tissue off gently.

Using fingers, rinse neck and face thoroughly with lukewarm water.

Then splash neck and face 30 times with cool water.

Dry neck and face.

Apply dry-skin cream (a rich lubricating one) liberally to neck and face for 5 to 15 minutes. (If you have 15 minutes, either take a bath or just relax and give yourself a massage.)

Then tissue off gently.

Using fingers, rinse neck and face thoroughly with lukewarm water.

Splash neck and face 30 times with cool water.

Dry neck and face.

Apply moisturizer liberally to neck and face.

Blot gently with tissue.

If you wish, give yourself a 2, 10 or 18 minute facial pick-up in the afternoon or before a date.

NOTE: Combination Skin can repeat morning schedule in a few hours if oiliness is present. Omit complexion brush, use fingers to lather soap on.

Oily Skin-Care Program

Morning

ALWAYS WASH HANDS BEFORE TOUCHING FACE.

Cleanse neck and face with mild complexion soap, use fingers to lather on, use natural-bristle complexion brush gently.

Using fingers, rinse off thoroughly with lukewarm water.

Then splash neck and face 30 times with cold water.

Dry neck and face.

Apply moisturizer liberally to neck and face.

Blot gently with tissue.

Repeat in a few hours omitting complexion brush and using a cleanser before the soap if you have make-up on.

If oiliness reappears in a few hours, repeat.

Evening

ALWAYS WASH HANDS BEFORE TOUCHING FACE.

Cleanse neck and face with whatever cleanser you prefer.

Tissue off gently.

Using fingers, rinse neck and face thoroughly with lukewarm water.

Cleanse neck and face with a mild complexion soap, use fingers to lather on.

Using fingers, rinse off thoroughly with lukewarm water.

Then splash neck and face 30 times with cold water.

*(Apply all-purpose skin cream to neck and face. Massage for 5 to 10 minutes. Tissue off. Using fingers, rinse neck and face thoroughly with lukewarm water. Then splash neck and face 30 times with cold water.)

Dry neck and face.

Blot gently with tissue.

If in the afternoon, or early evening, your face becomes oily, give yourself a facial pick-up. Repeat in a few hours if oiliness reappears.

Try to use a mask three times a week. (Do not apply near eye area.)

Try to change make-up every 4 hours if possible.

*2 to 3 times a week, use an all-purpose face cream. If over 30, try to use daily.

Combination Skin-Care Program

Follow the dry-skin program.

If oiliness is present, repeat the dry-skin morning program in a few hours. Omit the use of a complexion brush this time.

Sensitive Skin-Care Program

Follow the dry-skin program. Use hypo-allergic, non-perfumed products.

If your skin becomes irritated or "flares up", check with a dermatologist immediately.

How To Give Yourself A Massage

A massage for 5 to 10 minutes is helpful once or twice a week; once a day is good; 3 times a day ideal. Careful attention to correct finger movements is essential. Use a mirror to assure this.

With hair pinned or pulled back (a cotton headband launders easily), with plenty of oil or cream lubricant on neck and face (so you are massaging, not stretching), use both hands in a balanced action. Featherlight fingertips should slip lightly over neck and face, even for deep furrows and heavy wrinkles. Always up and out! Never rub hard, never pull downward on neck and face, never use heavy strokes, never pat, never slap or use force on the delicate structure or muscles of your neck and face.

Do carefully and correctly to get full benefits. Always up and out across lines so not to encourage sagging.

NECK MASSAGE

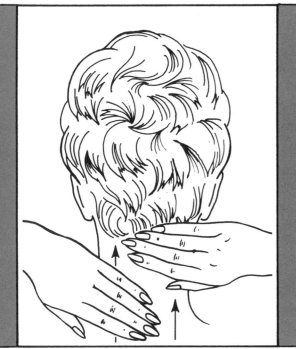

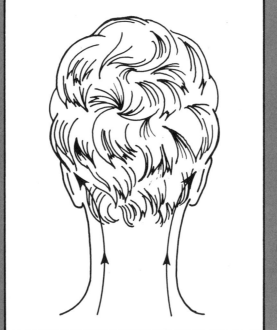

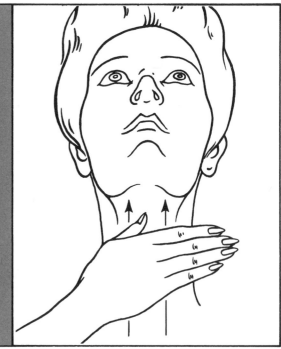

Use both hands. Reach over shoulders and down as far as possible, along spinal column, to the "dowager's hump." With featherlightness, fingers should slip up to the hairline. Do 3 times.

Then place palms on sides of back of neck and lightly slip up to ear. Do 3 times.

Place palm of hand at base of neck. Slip palm lightly up to chin. Do 3 times.

Morning	**Evening**

FACE MASSAGE

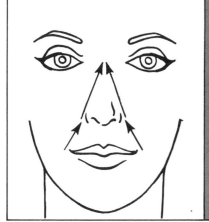 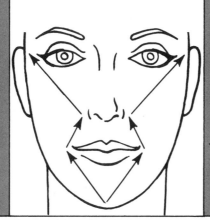 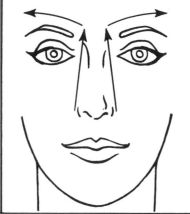 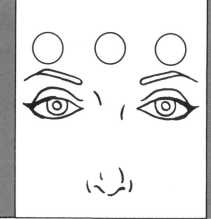

Slip fingertips from lip corner up to side of nose and up to bridge of nose where fingertips meet. Lift fingers from face. Do 3 times.

From chin, slip fingertips up to lip corner, up laugh line to nose, and then out to the upper part of the ear. Lift fingers from face. Do 3 times.

Place fingertips at base of nose, slip fingertips upward along nose and then out toward temple. Lift fingers from face. Do 3 times.

Make circles about the size of quarters over brow, moving always up and out toward hairline. Do 3 times.

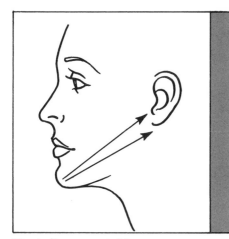 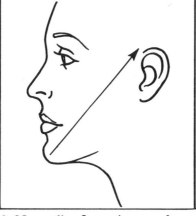 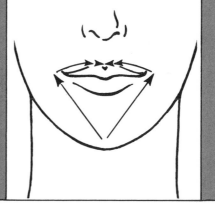 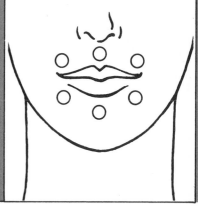

Rest elbows on table.

1. Slip featherlight fingertips up from chin to ear lobe. Lift fingers from face.

2. Now slip fingertips up from chin to middle of ear. Lift fingers from face.

3. Now slip fingertips up from chin to top of ear. Lift fingers from face.

Always so light you barely feel it.

Always up and out (NEVER DOWN). Do 3 times.

Start at chin, slip fingertips up to corners of mouth (lips).

Then around the upper lip to cupid's bow.

Press the two ridges of the bow together. Lift fingers from face. Do 3 times.

Lightly slip fingertips in little circles (about ½″ in diameter) around your lips as shown. Do once.

15

Masks

There are masks for oily, dry, and aging skins to stimulate, to give a temporary tightening and glow. They refresh, revitalize. Five minutes will usually produce an evident pick-up, though some masks need longer. For oily skin try to use a mask 3 times a week. For dry skin once a week is sufficient. Read all labels carefully and choose correctly for your needs.

Regular mask—all strengths and kinds; stimulates, tightens, gives a temporary glow.

Smoothing mask—concentrates on texture; refines and softens; may contain emollients to help revive dry skin.

Bracing mask—tightens pores, stimulates skin.

Medicated mask—aids dull disturbed skins.

Here's what to do.

Before you apply mask:

Pin hair back and use a headband (cotton preferred for easy laundering). Apply cleanser to neck and face. Tissue off. Using fingers, rinse neck and face thoroughly with lukewarm water. Then splash neck and face 30 times with lukewarm water. Dry neck and face. Gently dot on moisturizer, eye cream or oil to eye area.

Applying mask:

Be careful to avoid hairline and eye area, leave on, then remove, all as directed.

After mask removal:

Using fingers, rinse neck and face thoroughly with lukewarm water. Splash neck and face 30 times with cool water (dry skin), cold water (oily skin). Dry neck and face. *For oily skin,* apply moisturizer to neck and face. Blot gently with tissue. *For dry or combination skin,* apply dry-skin cream to neck and face for 5 to 15 minutes (give yourself a massage if you have time). Tissue off. Rinse neck and face thoroughly with lukewarm water. Splash neck and face 30 times with cool water. Dry neck and face. Apply moisturizer to neck and face. Blot gently with tissue.

You Can Make Your Own Mask

For oily skin many specialists say it's hard to find a better mask than this. It's simple and homemade.

Beat 2 egg whites until stiff. Apply to neck and face always up and out. Allow to dry for a few minutes, then rinse off thoroughly. Remove as directed in "After mask removal". Use mask 3 times a week on oily skin.

For dry skin try this.

Moisten oatmeal with water to a pasty consistency. Using fingers, apply to neck and face, always up and out. Let dry for 5 minutes (relax with feet up or take a soothing bath). Rinse off thoroughly. Remove as directed in "After mask removal". Use mask once a week on dry skin, if you wish.

2- to 30-Minute Facial Pick-ups

If you wish to change your make-up or get a quick lift before going out, try one of the following facial pick-ups.

2-Minute Facial Pick-up

1. Apply cleanser to neck and face.
2. Clean off.
3. Using fingers, rinse neck and face thoroughly with lukewarm water.
4. Then splash neck and face 30 times with cool water (dry skin), cold water (oily skin).
5. Dry neck and face.
6. Apply moisturizer to neck and face.
7. Blot gently with tissue.

6-Minute Facial Pick-up

Follow the first five steps of the 2-Minute Facial Pick-up. Then: For 5 minutes, apply mask best suited to your skin type. Leave on and then take off as directed for the product.

Using fingers, rinse neck and face thoroughly with lukewarm water.

Then splash neck and face 30 times with cool water (dry skin), cold water (oily skin).

Dry neck and face.

Apply moisturizer to neck and face.

Blot gently with tissue.

10-Minute Facial Pick-up

Follow the first five steps of the 2-Minute Facial Pick-up. Then: Apply skin cream to neck and face liberally, take a quick bath, or simply elevate your feet and relax for 5 minutes.

Then tissue cream off.

Using fingers, rinse neck and face thoroughly with lukewarm water.

Then splash neck and face 30 times with cool water (dry skin), cold water (oily skin).

Dry neck and face.

Apply moisturizer to neck and face.

Blot gently with tissue.

18-Minute Facial Pick-up

Follow the first five steps of the 2-Minute Facial Pick-up. Then:

Apply skin cream to neck and face liberally.

Give yourself a 5-minute massage.

Then relax (cream still on) with feet elevated, or take a quick shower or bath.

Tissue cream off.

Using fingers, rinse neck and face thoroughly with lukewarm water.

Then splash neck and face 30 times with cool water (dry skin), cold water (oily skin).

Apply moisturizer to neck and face.

Blot gently with tissue.

30-Minute Facial Pick-up

Follow the first five steps of the 2-Minute Facial Pick-up. Then:

Apply skin cream to neck and face liberally.

Give yourself a 5-minute massage.

Then relax (cream still on) with feet elevated, or take a 5-minute shower or bath.

Tissue cream off.

Using fingers, rinse neck and face thoroughly with lukewarm water.

Then splash neck and face 30 times with cool water (dry skin), cold water (oily skin).

Apply a 5-minute mask to neck and face.

Take off mask.

Using fingers, rinse neck and face thoroughly with lukewarm water.

Then splash neck and face 30 times with cool water (dry skin), cold water (oily skin).

Dry neck and face.

Apply moisturizer to neck and face.

Blot gently with tissue.

Other Facial-Care

Along with the meticulous care of your skin, attention should be given to all other facial features. Do not neglect any part of your face. Make sure you care for:

Teeth:

A smile can be one of your best beauty points. Don't mar it with missing, nonwhite, protruding, or irregular teeth. An improper bite may hinder digestion of food, keep you from receiving full benefit from food nutritionally. And missing teeth can change the contour of your face. So seek proper dental care, get a regular checkup and cleaning. If you have protruding or irregular teeth, it may be possible to correct them quite dramatically. Ask the advice of several orthodontists and find out what can be done. It is recommended that you use a toothpaste with fluoride and a natural-bristle toothbrush. Have your dentist suggest a proper-texture bristle for you, and get his advice on brushing.

Lips:

Use lip gloss, vaseline or moisturizer to keep lips from drying, cracking, or looking parched. Do lip exercises for supple lips. Try to keep lip corners up. Never pull down or tighten mouth corners. Don't press lips together.

Eyes:

Have your eye doctor check your eyes regularly. If you need (or wear) glasses, use them to avoid eyestrain. Strain and fatigue cause squinting, and squinting causes lines. Maintain proper distance and proper lighting while watching TV (always have a light on in the room). Make sure you have adequate light when reading or using your eyes. Use sun glasses to avoid excessive sun glare. Buy the best available (don't use plastic). Do eye exercises daily. Use eye lotion or drops regularly. Apply lots of moisturizer to the areas around the eyes. Be very careful not to rub under eyes. Dot on creams etc., with fingertips, and do not get too close to the eye.

Eyelashes:

Always remove all make-up from eyelashes each night. Apply vaseline (or any other excellent commercial preparation). Tissue off. Apply more vaseline. Tissue off again. If you wish to leave a little vaseline on, it may help to promote thickness and growth.

Eyebrows:

Brush brows daily with a clean mascara brush or a natural-bristle brush combined with a comb at the other end. Backstroke from the highest point, then from the outer end of brow, then brush back and comb into place. Use vaseline at night to train and keep in place. Tweeze (pluck) regularly for correct proportion, so the brows frame and set off the eyes. No stray hairs should remain.

Pluck your brows to suit your face. Be careful, for every hair counts. Try not to touch the top line itself (but do take out strays). Pluck from underneath. Here are a few basic principles:

The beginning (1) and ending (3) of the eyebrow should be the same level, *(3) never lower than (1)*.

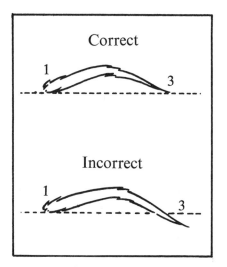

Experiment carefully until you find your best look.

Oval face:

The inner end of the eyebrow should begin immediately above the inner corner of the eye, its arch (highest peak) ending at the end of iris (when looking straight ahead), then tapering to end where the outside corner of the eye and the edge of the nostril indicate (use a ruler for this purpose as shown).

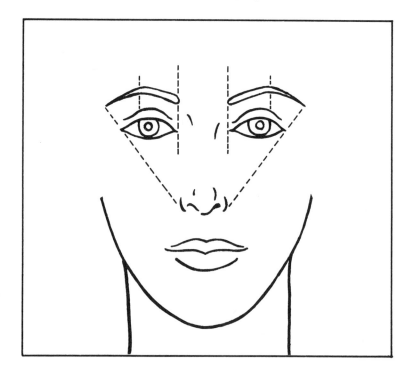

Narrow face:

Shorten length of eyebrow.

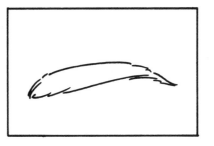

Broad face:

Extend length of eyebrow well to the side.

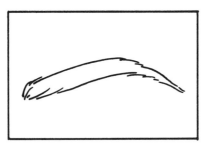

Round, plump faces:

Need angularity to eyebrow.

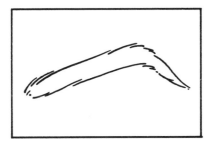

Close-set eyes, small features:

Pluck eyebrows farther apart than the inner corners (1) of the eyes.

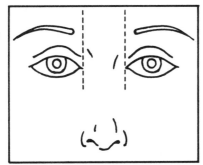

Narrow forehead:

Start eyebrow slightly farther out than the inner corner of the eye (1). The arch (2) should be beyond the iris. The distance from end of arch (2) and end of brow (3) should be ½ that from start of brow (1) to arch (2).

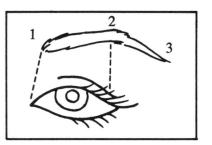

Wide forehead:

Start brow closer to nose. Extend it beyond inner corner of the eye (1). The arch (2) should be over the outer edge of the iris. The distance from (2) to (3) should be nearly the same length as the distance from (1) to (2).

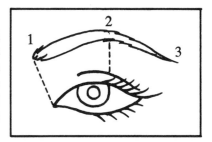

Forehead same width as jaw:

Start brow directly over inner corner of the eye (1). The arch (2) should be over the outer edge of the iris. The distance from (2) to (3) should be almost as long as from (1) to (2).

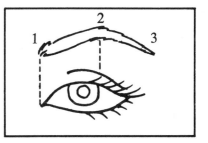

Skin Problems

No one's skin is perfect and problems frequently exist or occur.

Coarse Texture and Drying Due to Sun: Do not expose the face and neck to long periods of direct sun. This dries the skin and produces early wrinkles, prematurely ages the skin. Wear a broad-brimmed hat to shade the neck and face. Apply sun-screening lotion liberally, repeat fresh amounts at regular intervals. (And if in excessive sun glare, wear the best sun glasses you can afford. Squinting, too, causes wrinkles.)

Freckles: Freckles are caused by small areas of melanin pigment in the epidermis. They usually fade somewhat in winter, become more prominent in summer sun. Protect yourself from the sun and use a covering make-up to minimize the freckles' appearance.

Unwanted Hair: The root of each hair is embedded at the bottom of a microscopic shaft, or follicle. The follicle is a downgrowth of the layers of skin, and the hair that grows from it is a special form of the skin itself. And it needs good skin care. But excess facial hair is considered unsightly and unwanted. Several methods are used to camouflage and/or remove it.

Tweezing: Tweezing or plucking unwanted facial hair has no adverse effect, though it is somewhat displeasing. Usually the hair returns in 2 to 12 weeks.

Bleaching: Seek out any of the several good bleaches on the market and use as directed.

Electrolysis: Facial hair can be removed safely by electrolysis. This is a most effective and lasting method, but is not to be done except by a trained, fully-licensed, and experienced electrologist. A fine wire needle is introduced into the opening of each follicle, pushed down to the hair root, and an electric current is transmitted down the needle to destroy the root and loosen the hair for removal. When done correctly, there are no scars, no regrowth (and one experiences at most a very slight burning sensation).

Chemical Depilatories: Depilatories work by softening and dissolving the hair shaft. They do not destroy the root, so regrowth occurs, but results do last a little longer. Hair removal takes from 10 to 15 minutes. Depilatories should not be used on the face, however, unless the product's label so specifies. Many skin specialists do not recommend this method for the face.

Abrasives, Shaving, and Waxing are not recommended for the face.

Acne; Blackheads; Whiteheads; Pimples: Acne is a disorder of the skin glands, not contagious, characterized by the interaction of one's own hormones, sebaceous glands, and bacteria. It is most common to teen-agers (authorities say that more than 80% of teen-agers get acne in some degree). Between the ages of 12 and 20, principally, certain glands speed up the production of male and female hormones; these stimulate the oil glands in the skin to produce excess oil, the root of the trouble. Ordinarily the skin's sebaceous glands send up small amounts of oil to soften and protect the skin. When overstimulated, however, they enlarge, send up too much

FORMATION OF PIMPLES

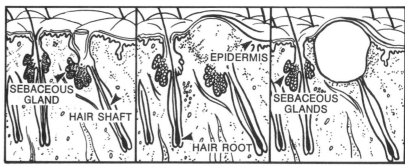

BLACKHEAD   PUSTULE   CYST

sebum too frequently, and in the walls of the canals of supply, bacteria lurk. The bacteria produce enzymes which act on the sebum, or oil, and break it down into intensely irritating acids. Acne is the result. Acne is typified by spots, blemishes, pimples and eruptions of various kinds, primarily appearing on the forehead, cheeks, and chin. In adults the condition is an exception, but may sometimes come forth because of severe stress, emotional upset, change of climate, tension, worry, or excitement.

Hundreds of tiny oil sacs (sebaceous glands) are underneath the skin. These glands are attached to a follicle tube from which small and fragile hairs emerge. Usually oil from the sebaceous gland rises through the follicle tube to the skin surface, carrying with it skin debris and minute particles of body waste. This is called sebum. When the oil glands start overproducing oil, the skin becomes excessively oily. The sebum plugs up pores. When this sebum is exposed to air, it turns black (due to a chemical reaction with oxygen, NOT due to dirt) and is called a blackhead (comedo).

If sebum is not exposed to air but can be seen beneath the surface of the skin, it is called a whitehead (papule).

When bacteria cause infection in the follicle, the result is a pimple (pustule).

Washing 4 to 6 times a day with an antibacterial cleanser is very important to help control and remove excess oil, help reduce the bacteria growth, loosen and open comedones, and to produce a drying effect. Always rinse thoroughly with water after each washing. Make sure that everything that touches your skin is immaculate. Follow a daily exercise routine; eat three balanced, nutritionally-correct meals each day; get lots of sleep; drink plenty of water for regular elimination and other benefits; never scrub, rub, or pinch your face; change your pillow case daily.

It is also important to keep scalp oils and dandruff flakes (if you have any) from accumulating and getting onto your skin. So keep your hair and scalp clean. Washing your hair every day, every other day or every third day will not hurt (lather only once with a pure castile shampoo; follow with conditioner). Whether you wash your hair once a week or once a day depends on where you live and the type of hair you have. Just do not allow hair to get oily. Brushing 100 strokes daily with a genuine natural-bristle brush takes out dirt and scales (also adds shine, luster, stimulates circulation, and massages the scalp for healthy hair growth). Keep brush and comb clean.

Each person's problem is individual, but if serious acne develops at any age, consult a qualified dermatologist immediately, for much can now be done to prevent permanent scarring or pitting of the skin.

Rashes, Moles, Wens, Warts, Birthmarks, Pockmarks, Feature Changes, Lifts, etc. Never try to treat a serious skin problem at home. The risk of scarred, damaged or ruined skin is simply NOT worth it! See a dermatologist. Many do clinic-work with fees adjusted to financial ability, so the best care is not beyond your reach. Do use it. Do not prescribe for, nor attempt to cure any of these conditions yourself. You may start out with a minor problem, have it turn into a major one, perhaps even slow down favorable results by doing exactly the wrong thing.

Dermabrasion and skin peels can produce a smooth skin from one otherwise pockmarked and rough. Consult a qualified dermatologist to advise you.

Cosmetic surgery can correct any number of skin problems; can even effect nose, lip, or eyelid changes, lifts, and the correction of receding chins. Since this is not a book on surgical beauty methods, but a facial-care and exercise program, we shall not go into detail about this. If you're contemplating cosmetic surgery, *be sure you choose a competent plastic surgeon!* Know the man you're dealing with, or have him recommended by your doctor.

And here, money should not be an object.

Remember tampering with nature's expression areas can be dangerous. So be very careful, know what to expect both before and after cosmetic surgery, but do not be frightened of it. It can offer quite marvelous results, even related beneficial psychological changes.

Good Eating Habits For A Radiant Complexion

The foods we eat are a key factor in the maintenance of a radiant complexion. A daily balance of the 5 basic food groups is essential nutritionally for good cell reproduction and cell growth. So forget starvation diets (you can eat a lot and keep calories low if you know what you are doing), forget food fads; don't eat just one food group even if it is the "in" thing to do.

If you are eating a proper balance of these 5 basic food groups daily, and in variety, supplementary vitamins and minerals usually will not be needed. Maintain sensible eating habits. The amount of food your body requires depends on your age, size, sex, and the work you do. If dieting, don't cut out, but cut down. Size of helpings should be determined by energy needs. If you are on a diet, you're eating less so it is now more important than ever that you eat correctly to get all the vitamins and minerals your body requires to function healthfully.

Prepare your food carefully; don't expose it for long periods; do not overcook; do cook and serve immediately; use only what you need to avoid leftovers. Nutritious, inexpensive meals can be aromatic, eye-appealing, and delicious. Remember that no single food can provide all the nutrients your complexion and your body need; variety, combination, preparation, and balance are of the utmost importance, so evaluate your menus and plan for each week judiciously.

Good nutrition is vital to physical and emotional well-being. We need it for growth, for the maintenance and repair of body cells and tissues, and for energy production. All the nutrients we require can be found in "everyday" foods, available inexpensively the year 'round, as long as we combine and select from the 5 basic food groups, keep variety in our eating, and properly cook what we eat.

Except for a decrease in calories for those over 60, authorities now agree their nutrient requirements are the same as for people of middle age. Greater care, therefore, must be used in the selection of food—so, though there is less food, it's still as nutritious.

(It should be noted that special foods are available for those with special problems, from chewing to dietetic restrictions and impaired gastrointestinal functions.)

The 5 basic food groups are:
Meat and Fish
Bread and Cereal
Vegetable
Fruit
Milk

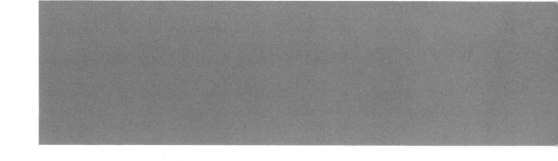

MEAT AND FISH GROUP: (poultry, meat, fish, eggs, dry beans, dry peas, and nuts).

A 3-ounce serving of lean meat, poultry or fish without bone is the minimum adult daily serving. 2 servings or more for adults is fine. Larger servings may be needed for more active or growing persons. Smaller for children.

Alternative daily requirements are 2 eggs, 1 cup of dry beans, dry peas, or lentils; or four tablespoons of peanut butter.

Although a peanut butter sandwich does not seem as luxurious as a steak, it can accomplish about the same thing in the body. Spending money does not necessarily mean eating nutritiously.

BREAD AND CEREAL GROUP: (whole grained, enriched or restored).

A variety of four or more servings of the following is recommended daily:

1 slice of bread (equals 1 serving).

1 serving cold cereal, ready to eat.

½ to ¾ cup of cooked cereal or substitute, such as grits, corn meal, rice, rolled oats, spaghetti, macaroni, noodles, etc.

VEGETABLE GROUP: (often neglected, considered tasteless because of improper preparation).

Two or more servings daily is recommended of any of the following: broccoli, green pepper, sweet red pepper, carrots, chard, collards, cress, kale, spinach, sweet potatoes, turnip greens, winter squash, or any dark green or deep yellow vegetable.

FRUIT GROUP: (often neglected).

It is very important to have a good fruit source of Vitamin A* and one serving daily of a good fruit source of Vitamin C; or two servings of fair sources of both.

Good Source Vitamin A	Good Source Vitamin C	Fair Source Vitamins A or C
apricot	grapefruit or grapefruit juice	honeydew melon
cantaloupe	orange or orange juice	tangerine or
persimmon	cantaloupe	tangerine juice
pumpkin	guava	watermelon
tomato	mango	
	papaya	
	raw fresh strawberries	

*Vitamin A is stored in the body; 3 or 4 servings a week are adequate

MILK GROUP: (whole milk, skim-milk, evaporated milk, buttermilk, butter, cheese, ice cream).

Milk or some other dairy product is strongly recommended. Most authorities feel the minimum daily requirement for milk is:

Children:	3 to 4 cups (8 oz. to a cup)
Teen-agers:	4 or more cups
Adults, all ages:	2 cups
Pregnant women:	4 or more cups
Nursing mothers:	6 or more cups

Some quick reference equivalents are:

⅔ cup milk *or* 1″ cube cheddar cheese

⅓ cup milk *or* ½ cup cottage cheese

¼ cup milk *or* ½ cup ice cream

To summarize:

At the very least, do try to have the following every day.

3 slices of enriched or whole-wheat bread

1 helping of enriched cereal

at least one egg

1 helping of citrus fruit

1 helping of raw or cooked non-citrus fruit

1-2 pats of butter

2 green or yellow vegetables

1 potato or 1 helping of rice, macaroni, noodles, spaghetti, etc.

1 ounce of cheese

3-4 ounces of meat, poultry or fish

2 glasses of milk

And 3 to 5 glasses of water (bottled spring water recommended).

Facial
Exercises

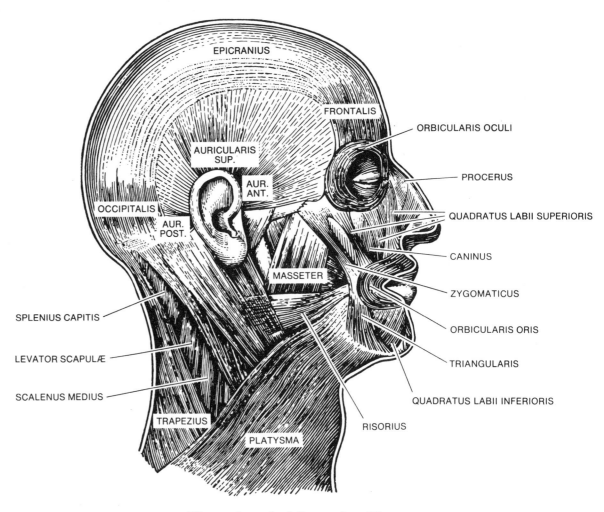

EPICRANIUS

FRONTALIS

ORBICULARIS OCULI

AURICULARIS SUP.

AUR. ANT.

PROCERUS

OCCIPITALIS

QUADRATUS LABII SUPERIORIS

AUR. POST.

CANINUS

MASSETER

ZYGOMATICUS

SPLENIUS CAPITIS

ORBICULARIS ORIS

LEVATOR SCAPULÆ

TRIANGULARIS

SCALENUS MEDIUS

QUADRATUS LABII INFERIORIS

TRAPEZIUS

RISORIUS

PLATYSMA

The various facial muscles. There are 14 major facial muscle groups

Why Facial Exercises?

Under the facial skin there are bones, blood vessels, connective tissue, fat, nerves, and muscles. The very contour of your face is determined by the bones of the skull, the muscle flesh underneath the skin, and by the muscles partly attached to the skin. You are only able to have facial movements in fact (lip movements, squinting, frowning), because the muscles attached to the inner skin exist. Once one grows up biologically, however, the muscles of the face start a downward trend, and skin elasticity starts to disappear. Sagging and lines appear.

Age Lines: Muscles attached to the inner skin weaken, fatten, or shrink if unexercised over the years. Thus the areas they control are potential targets for age lines, folds and furrows. But if the muscles are toned through exercise, they will have (as they *must* have) the elastic ability to regain their original size and shape after being stretched. The elastic quality of the skin and the muscles beneath it help determine firmness and smoothness. Youth's face is firm and smooth, but this need not be solely theirs if everyone's muscles are properly toned. And gaining good muscle control through exercise can help one correct the effects of the downward pull of gravity, help keep your skin elastic, firm, and tight. It will also help you counter the other type of lines *not* due to age: caused expression lines.

Lines Not Due To Age: Expression lines are formed by the habit of "setting" one's expression; using muscles to express various emotions too often and "holding" for too long a time. Even in late teens one may have them to some degree.

Of course you should have a mobile and responsive face, but don't constantly use and hold the same expression. You should not (for example) keep eyebrows raised for long periods of time. It may make you look silly or unattractive, but more importantly, it creates

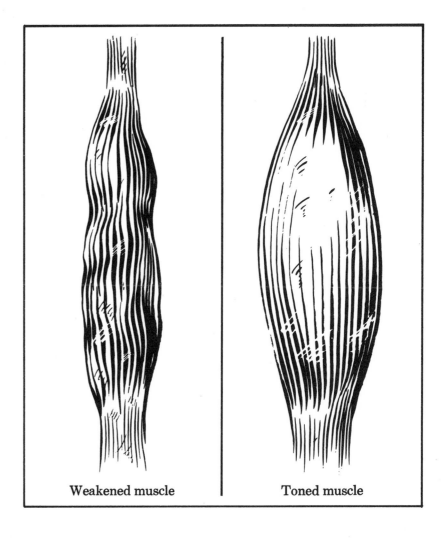

Weakened muscle   Toned muscle

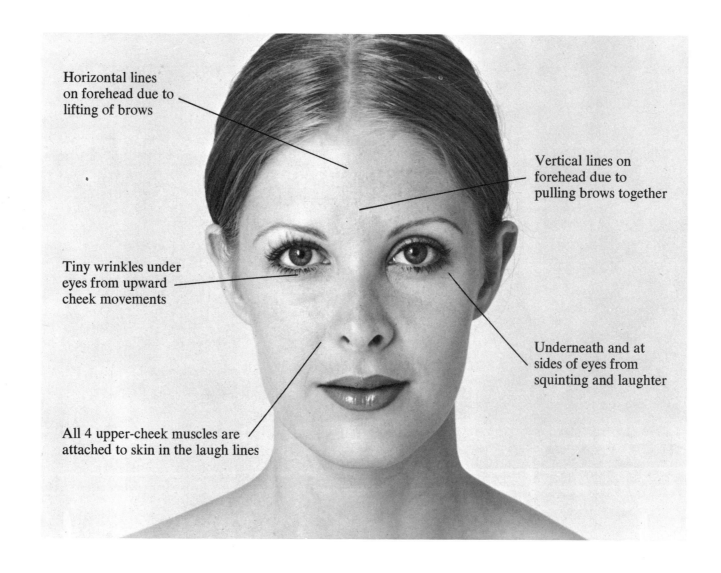

Horizontal lines on forehead due to lifting of brows

Vertical lines on forehead due to pulling brows together

Tiny wrinkles under eyes from upward cheek movements

Underneath and at sides of eyes from squinting and laughter

All 4 upper-cheek muscles are attached to skin in the laugh lines a line, or lines, where none should be. A frown sometimes appears on faces all day long. It becomes a habit, then a set expression with accompanying lines. (Most expression lines have nothing to do with aging.) The areas in which they are commonly found are shown on page 30. Correction or prevention comes with muscle control. It takes time, practice, proper care, and exercise. Muscle movements must be reversed and habitual expressions altered.

Facial radiance can keep expression lines, as from frowns, away. Expression lines are a reflection of your mental and emotional life. If you take an interest in things, in what is happening around you, you'll keep up to date. People will find you current and interesting. Your feelings about yourself will be positive and your face will project this. You'll have an inner glow, a ready smile, a joyful spirit, and a facial radiance. That constant frown will soon disappear!

Daily Facial Movements: So often people observe, then ask: "I have a mobile face, use it all day in ordinary facial movements; how are your exercises different from what I do each day . . . ?"

Ordinary daily facial movements use involuntary muscles for blinking, smiling, talking, and the like. The exercises offered here reach voluntary face muscles not normally used daily as well as involuntary muscles. These exercises, if followed correctly and consistently, will tone and help firm those long neglected muscles.

Myth and Misconception: Many people think facial exercises cause sagging, more lines, stretch the skin.

No. Proper exercising does not. On the contrary, if your facial muscles are not exercised, sagging and wrinkles will occur due to the weakening of muscles and the pull of gravity. Regular daily exercise helps prevent this, and maintains and rehabilitates skin elasticity. Don't be afraid to move your face. It is lack of movement and proper exercise that causes the problems.

Age Does Not Matter: You should begin exercising in your 20's to help prevent the formation of early lines and wrinkles.

Nor is it ever too late to start. If you have furrows or sagging lines, it is an indication of muscles not toned. *Start toning them today!*

Results: The time needed to see results varies with each individual and depends on age, the problem, whether the exercises and program are done correctly and regularly. Some women see improvement in a day, some in a few weeks, others in a few months. Consistency and attention to directions count.

The degree of result depends. The exercises won't do as much as a surgical face lift, but they (plus the face-care program) will help you look like you don't need one!

Exercise Properly: These exercises should be done in very-slow-motion. The importance of moving muscles slowly cannot be over-stressed. Best results come when individual muscle fibers are fully used. When you move a muscle *quickly,* gravity and momentum help, so you do not use all the muscle fibers (each muscle can contain from 3 to 165 fibers) and a portion of the muscle is unused, therefore, not exercised, and not receiving benefits. Do the exercises slowly with correct and careful attention to all directions.

Your Looks Are Up To You: If you worry about how you look now, or how you'll start to look—don't! Try the exercises on a regular basis and you'll find it's how you look afterwards that counts. Your looks are up to you, and your facial skin is only as firm as the muscle structure beneath it. So let's firm and tone these muscles (voluntary and involuntary) for a tight smooth face. Muscular collapse due to aging takes a long time. Why not take a few minutes each day to help prevent it?

Points to Remember

1. Do daily, if possible. Do some or all the exercises as your needs dictate. Order does not matter. Isolate your problem(s) or do the entire 6-Minute plan. Always wash hands before touching the face, make sure nails are clean.

2. Use a mirror while doing exercises so you can be sure you are doing them correctly. Correct positions are essential. Follow directions carefully and allow enough time for the exercises to work. Refer back to the directions regularly (after they are memorized) as a check that you are doing everything correctly. Some of the exercises take time to accomplish and cannot be done immediately. With some practice and attention to direction, you'll soon do them. If you need to use your fingers to help at first, gently do so.

3. Do anytime, anywhere (standing, sitting, in bed or bathtub).

4. Be relaxed as you exercise. Do each exercise evenly, smoothly, never jerkily, slowly, never fast. You MUST do exercises in *very-slow-motion.*

5. *Do not apply cream (or anything else) to your face while exercising. Face should be dry and free of everything.* Never use a machine in connection with these exercises, no massages and no facial manipulation while doing the exercises.

6. Breathe deeply and frequently as you exercise.

7. An occasional blemish may appear during the first week. Don't worry. It's due to the fresh flow of natural oil to tissues that haven't received it in a long time. The blemish will disappear after a week or so.

8. If you contemplate doing these exercises before or after surgery, or after injuries, or if you have high blood pressure or physical defects, show the exercises to your physician before beginning the program and ask his advice on your ability to do the program, how much of it, and at what rate of progress.

9. *Never strain.* If muscles tire, do not do more as you will not benefit. Do a little, consistently, for best results.

10. **Before you start the exercises,** if possible, cleanse neck and face, tissue off, rinse neck and face thoroughly with lukewarm water. Dry neck and face. To achieve best results use featherlike movements (no heavy fingers, no rubbing, never be harsh or hard on your face). Then do the exercises you wish to do.

When you finish exercising, wash your neck and face with soap (oily skin), with cleanser (dry or combination skin). Rinse thoroughly with lukewarm water.

For oily skin splash neck and face 30 times with cold water. Dry neck and face. Apply moisturizer and blot gently with tissue.

For dry, combination, or sensitive skin, dry face, apply dry-skin cream to neck and face for 5 to 10 minutes (give yourself a massage if you have time). Tissue off. Rinse thoroughly with lukewarm water. Splash neck and face 30 times with cool water. Dry neck and face. Apply moisturizer liberally to neck and face. Blot gently with tissue.

Sana-Facial-Exercises

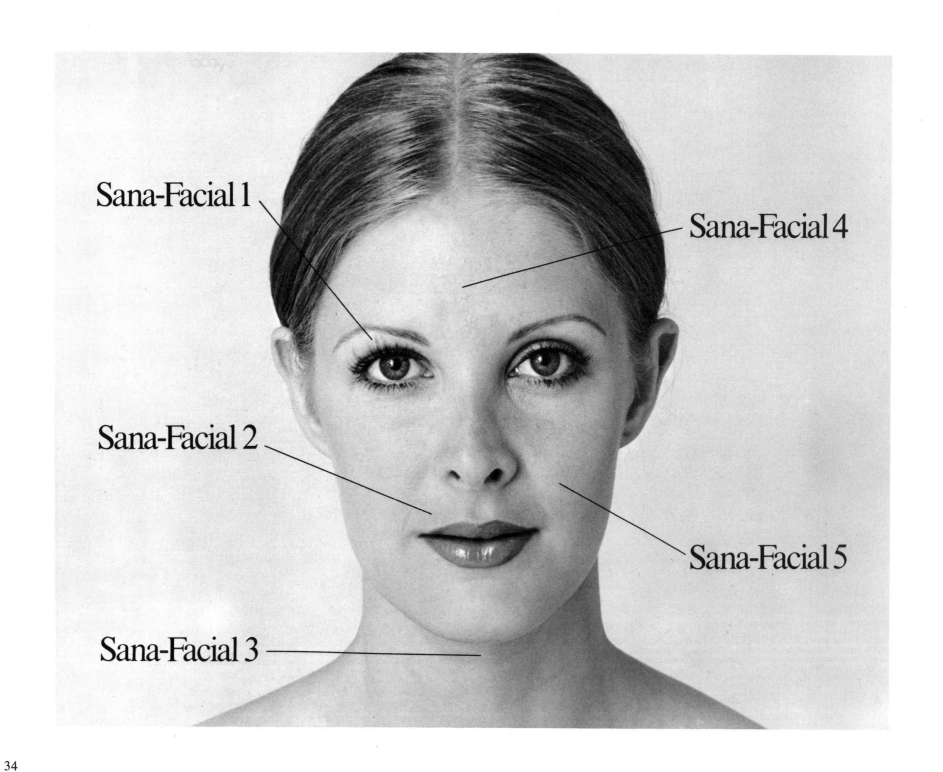

Sana-Facial 1

Sana-Facial 4

Sana-Facial 2

Sana-Facial 5

Sana-Facial 3

34

Sana-Facial 1

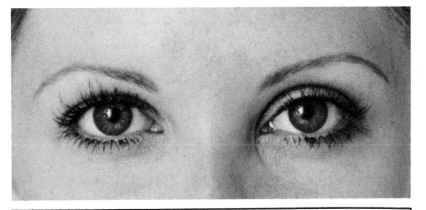

DROOPING
SAGGING
CROWS FEET
PUFFINESS
CIRCLES
LINES

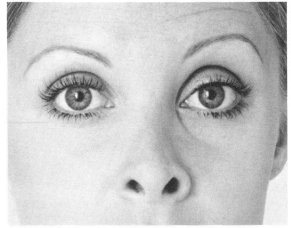

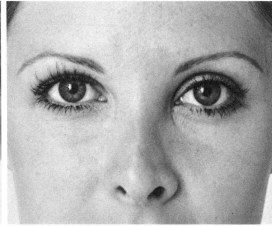

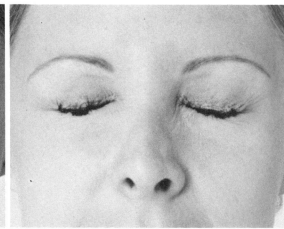

With eyes open, raise eyebrows to their highest possible position to the slow count of 1 and 2 and 3 and 4 and 5 and 6.

With eyebrows still raised blink 10 times.

Lower eyebrows to the count of 1 and 2 and 3 and 4 and 5 and 6.

Relax while counting 1 and 2 and 3.

Close eyes tightly while counting 1 and 2 and 3 and 4 and 5 and 6.

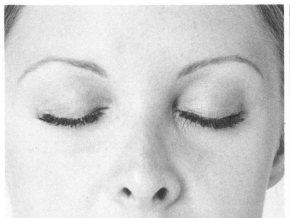

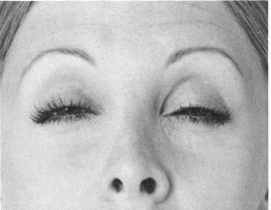

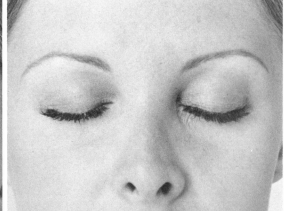

Stop pressing.
Leave eyes closed and relaxed while counting 1 and 2 and 3.

Open eyes. Blink 10 times.

Raise eyebrows. Raise lower eyelids.

Lower upper eyelids (squinting—lids centered).

Hold while counting 1 and 2 and 3 and 4 and 5 and 6. Then lower eyebrows.

Close eyes.
Relax while counting 1 and 2 and 3.

Open eyes. Blink 10 times.

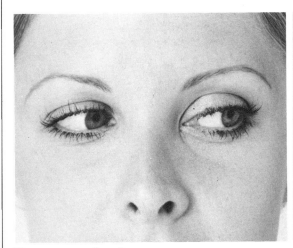

Do not move head.

Look right as far as you can.

Hold while counting 1 and 2 and 3 and 4 and 5 and 6.

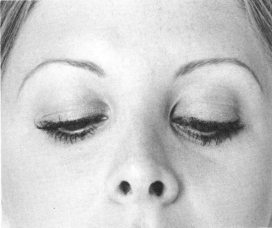

Then look down as far as you can.

Hold while counting 1 and 2 and 3 and 4 and 5 and 6.

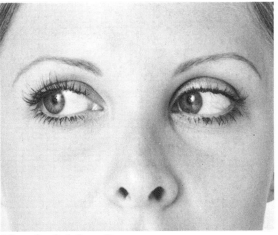

Then look left as far as you can.

Hold while counting 1 and 2 and 3 and 4 and 5 and 6.

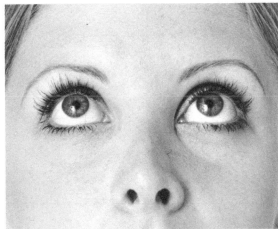

Then look up as far as you can.

Hold while counting 1 and 2 and 3 and 4 and 5 and 6.

Return eyes to normal front position.

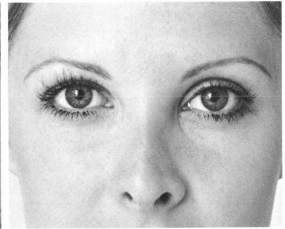

Relax, blinking eyes while counting 1 and 2 and 3.

Sana-Facial 1
Do 1 Time

EYE STRAIN
PUFFINESS
LOWER EYELIDS

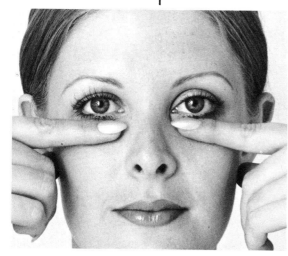

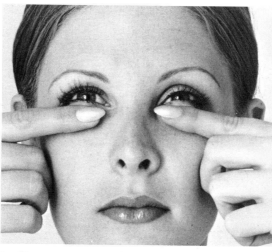

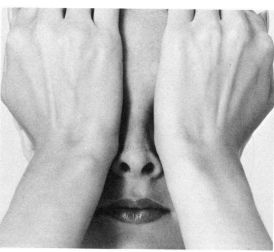

Place index fingers over lower eyelids and lower part of eyes.

Close eyes while counting 1 and 2 and 3 and 4 and 5 and 6.

Apply pressure gently upward 3 times and then downward 3 times. Do not allow nails to touch skin.

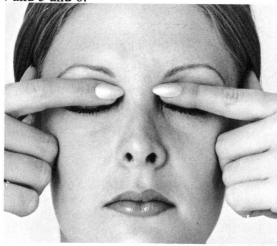

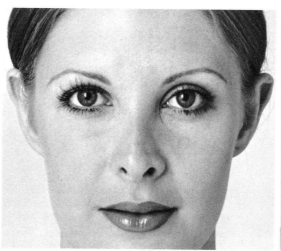

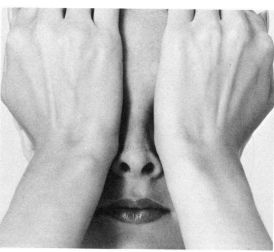

Next place index fingers over closed eyes.

Apply gentle inward pressure to the closed eyelids while counting 1 and 2 and 3 and 4 and 5 and 6. Remove fingers.

Relax while counting 1 and 2 and 3.
Open eyes. Blink several times.

Cup eyes with palms of hands.
Do not put pressure on eyeballs.
Allow no light in. Hold while counting to 60.

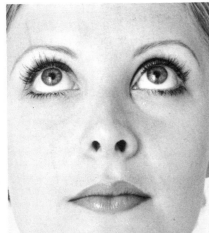

Do not move head. Look up as far as you can.

Hold while counting 1 and 2 and 3 and 4 and 5 and 6.

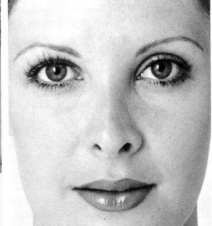

Return eyes to normal front position.

Relax, blinking eyes while counting 1 and 2 and 3.

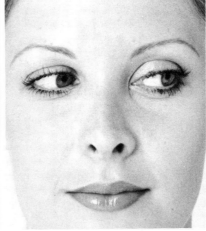

With head motionless, look right as far as you can.

Hold while counting 1 and 2 and 3 and 4 and 5 and 6.

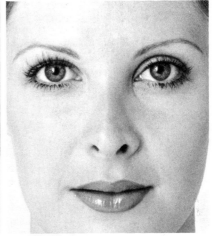

Return eyes to normal front position.

Relax, blinking eyes while count- 1 and 2 and 3.

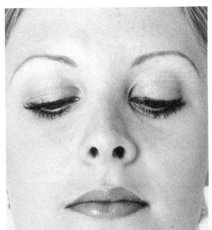

With head motionless, look down as far as you can.

Hold while counting 1 and 2 and 3 and 4 and 5 and 6.

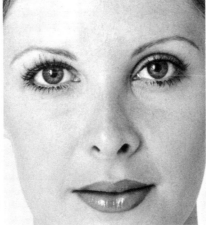

Return eyes to normal front position.

Relax, blinking eyes while counting 1 and 2 and 3.

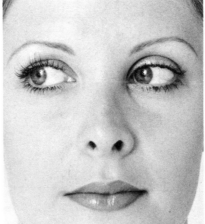

With head motionless, look left as far as you can.

Hold while counting 1 and 2 and 3 and 4 and 5 and 6.

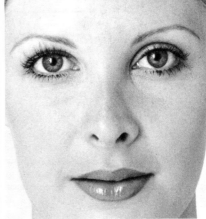

Return eyes to normal front position.

Relax, blinking eyes while count- ing 1 and 2 and 3.

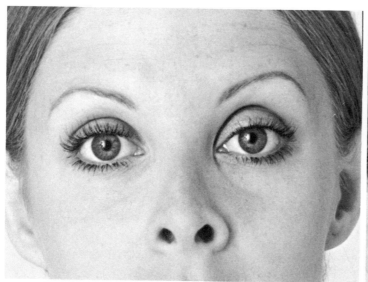

Open eyes as wide as possible.

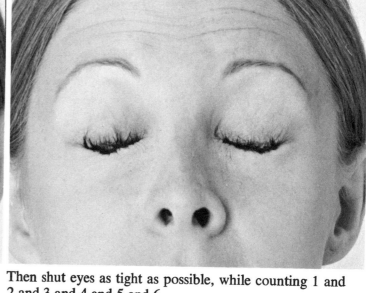

Then shut eyes as tight as possible, while counting 1 and 2 and 3 and 4 and 5 and 6.

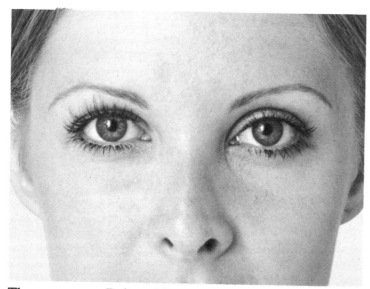

Then open eyes. Relax while counting 1 and 2 and 3.

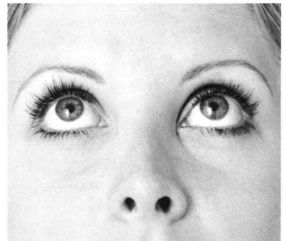

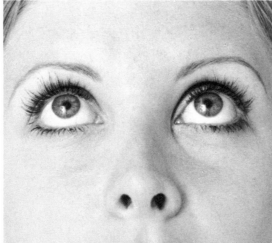

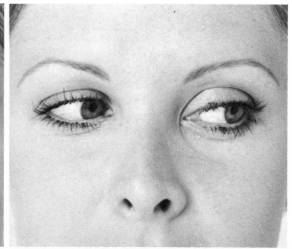

Keep head motionless. Look left as far as you can. Hold position. Blink eyes while counting 1 and 2 and 3 and 4 and 5 and 6.

Then look up and over to the right as far as you can making a half circle with your eyes. Hold position. Blink eyes while counting 1 and 2 and 3 and 4 and 5 and 6.

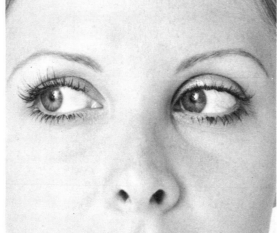

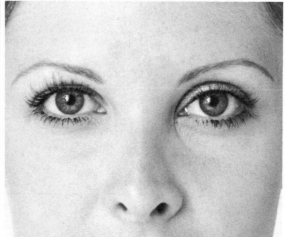

Then look up and over to the right as far as you can making a half circle with your eyes. Hold position. Blink eyes while counting 1 and 2 and 3 and 4 and 5 and 6.

Then return eyes to front. Blink eyes while counting 1 and 2 and 3 and 4 and 5 and 6.

Repeat making a lower half circle.

Sana-Facial 2

UPPER LIP
LOWER LIP
POUCHES
SIDES OF MOUTH
UPPER CHIN

Sana-Facial 2

Do 1 Time | LIPS

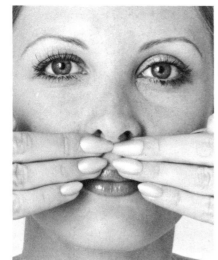

Place fingers as shown.

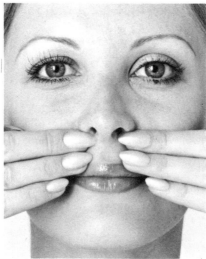

Pull outward.

Hold while counting 1 and 2 and 3 and 4 and 5 and 6.

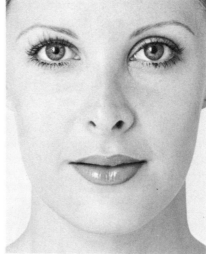

Stop pulling. Remove fingers.

Relax while counting 1 and 2 and 3.

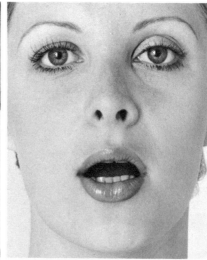

Open mouth slightly, teeth parted about ¼ inch.

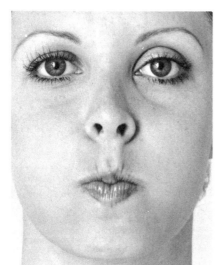

Take a deep breath.

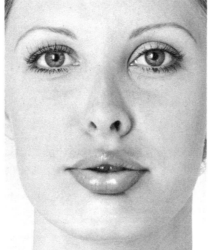

Exhale by blowing through lips so they flutter.

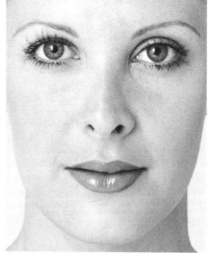

Relax while counting 1 and 2 and 3.

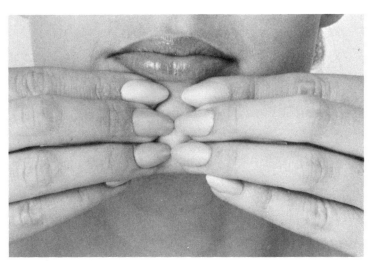

Place fingers as shown.

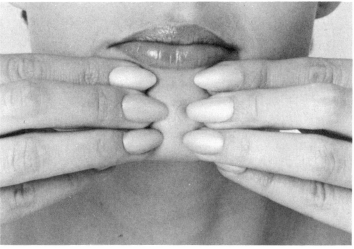

Pull outward.
(Do not use mouth to help pull chin outward.)
Hold while counting 1 and 2 and 3 and 4 and 5 and 6.
Stop pulling.

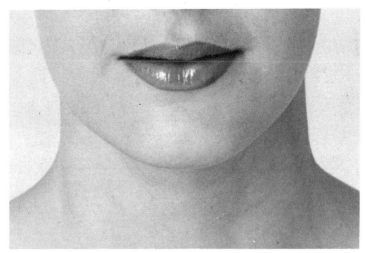

Remove fingers.
Relax while counting 1 and 2 and 3.

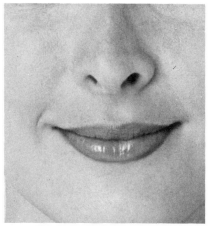

Keep lips and teeth together.

Smile with mouth closed lifting mouth corners as high as possible.

(No lines should appear around eyes.) Hold while counting 1 and 2 and 3 and 4 and 5 and 6.

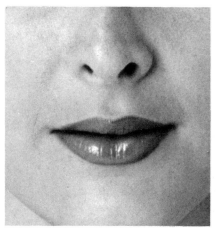

Stop smiling.

Relax while counting 1 and 2 and 3.

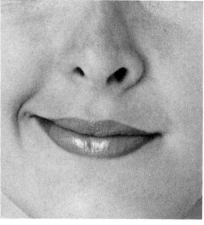

Lift left mouth corner as high as you can.

Hold while counting 1 and 2 and 3 and 4 and 5 and 6.

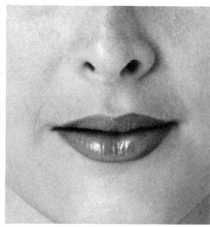

Then lower left mouth corner.

Relax while counting 1 and 2 and 3.

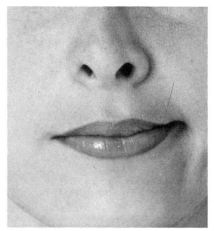

Lift right mouth corner as high as you can.

Hold while counting 1 and 2 and 3 and 4 and 5 and 6.

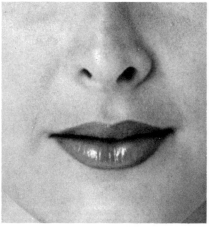

Then lower right mouth corner.

Relax while counting 1 and 2 and 3.

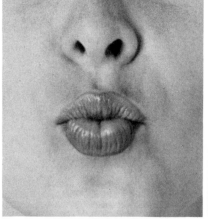

Keep lips together.

Push lips out (pucker).

Hold while counting 1 and 2 and 3 and 4 and 5 and 6.

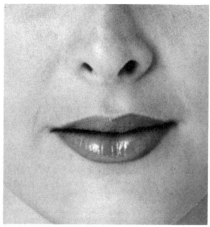

Relax mouth.

Then count 1 and 2 and 3.

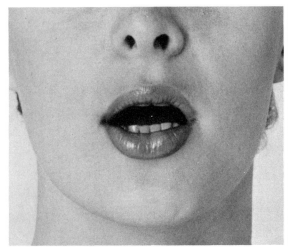

Open mouth, teeth 1 inch apart.

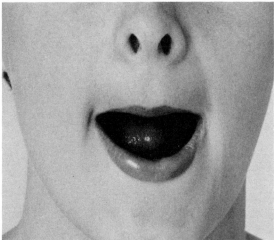

Keep lower lip and teeth in this position as you move upper lip downward as far as you can. Hold while counting 1 and 2 and 3 and 4 and 5 and 6.

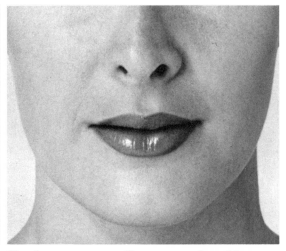

Slowly return upper lip to normal position.

Close mouth.

Relax while counting 1 and 2 and 3.

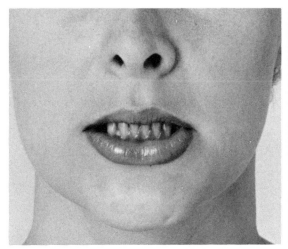

Lips lightly parted, teeth together, push lower lip downward so lower teeth can be seen.

Hold while counting 1 and 2 and 3 and 4 and 5 and 6.

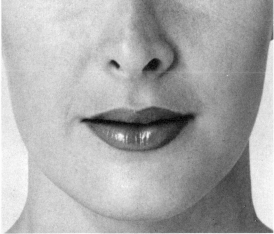

Close mouth.

Relax while counting 1 and 2 and 3.

47

Sana-Facial 2

Do 1 Time

LOWER LIP
UPPER CHIN
FURROWS

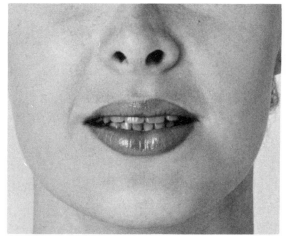

Open mouth.
Keep teeth together.

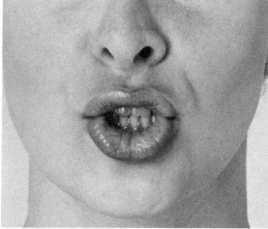

Form an O with lips as you push lips outward letting lips curl backward.
Hold while counting 1 and 2 and 3 and 4 and 5 and 6.

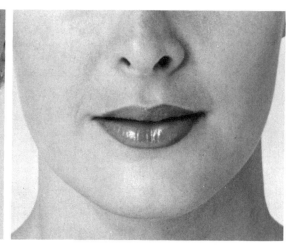

Close mouth.
Relax while counting 1 and 2 and 3.

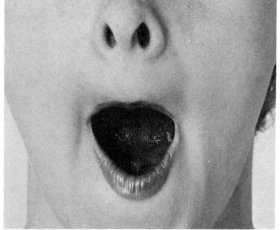

Open mouth and teeth.
Pull lips into mouth over teeth as far as you can.
Hold while counting 1 and 2 and 3 and 4 and 5 and 6.

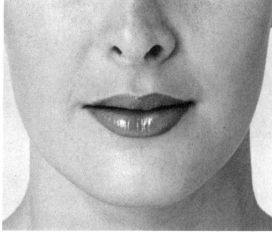

Close mouth.
Relax lips while counting 1 and 2 and 3.

Sana-Facial 3

UNDER CHIN

DOUBLE CHIN

NECK

Sana-Facial 3
Do 1 Time

DOUBLE CHIN
NECK

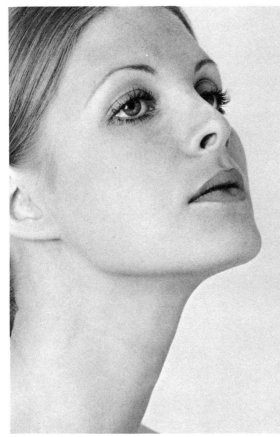

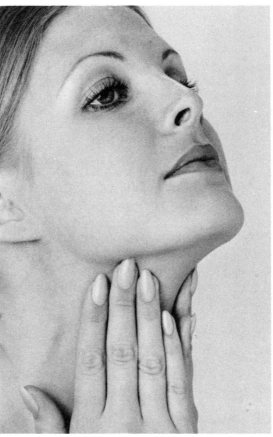

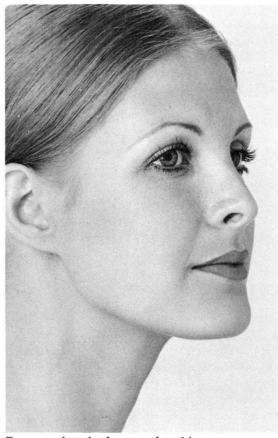

Raise chin as far as you can. Move head only.

(Do not move neck or body.) Keep teeth closed, lips together, mouth immobile.

Now push tip of tongue straight ahead against teeth—keep pushing as you hold.

Try to push lower chin up toward mouth.

Hold while counting 1 and 2 and 3 and 4 and 5 and 6.

Relax *tongue* while counting 1 and 2 and 3.

Keep teeth and mouth closed.

Press tip of tongue against lower teeth.

With fingers of each hand find hollows under chin and press.

Hold while counting 1 and 2 and 3 and 4 and 5 and 6.

Now press tip of tongue against upper teeth while counting 1 and 2 and 3 and 4 and 5 and 6.

Next press top of tongue straight ahead against teeth while counting 1 and 2 and 3 and 4 and 5 and 6.

Remove thumbs from under chin.

Lower chin to normal position.

Relax while counting 1 and 2 and 3.

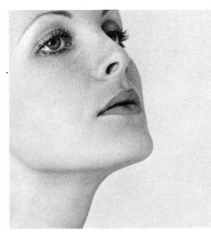

Raise chin as far as you can.
Move head only. *(Do not move neck or body.)*

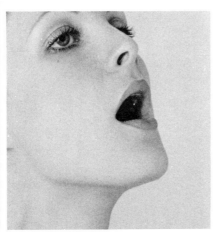

Slowly open mouth as wide as possible while counting 1 and 2 and 3 and 4 and 5 and 6.

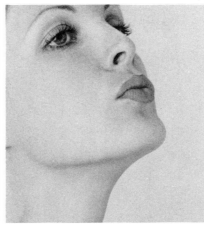

Close mouth.
Slowly push lips outward to a pucker, lips curling backward, while counting 1 and 2 and 3 and 4 and 5 and 6. Relax lips.

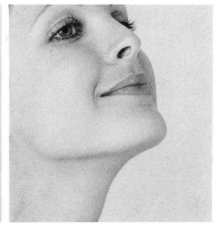

Then smile, keeping mouth closed, while counting 1 and 2 and 3 and 4 and 5 and 6.
Stop smiling.

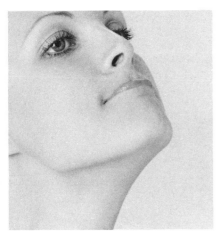

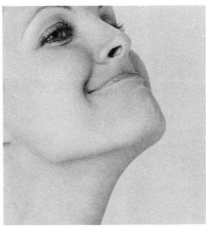

Hold while counting 1 and 2 and 3 and 4 and 5 and 6.

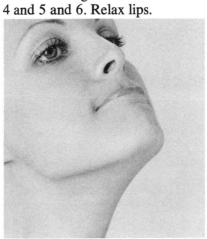

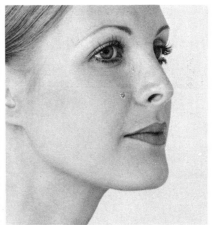

Lower chin to normal position.
Relax while counting 1 and 2 and 3.

Sana-Facial 3

Do 1 Time | NECK

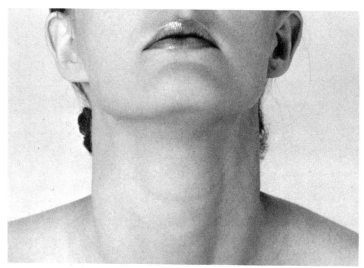

Pull shoulders down as you look up, raising chin as high as possible.

Hold while counting 1 and 2 and 3 and 4 and 5 and 6.

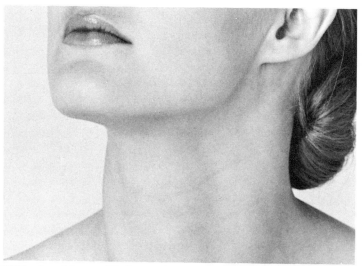

With shoulders still down look over shoulder as far as you can.

Hold while counting 1 and 2 and 3 and 4 and 5 and 6.

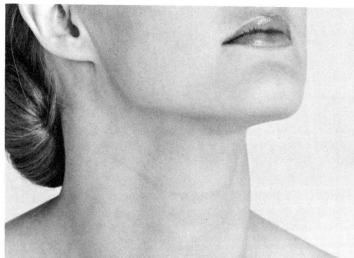

With shoulders still down look over opposite shoulder as far as you can.

Hold while counting 1 and 2 and 3 and 4 and 5 and 6.

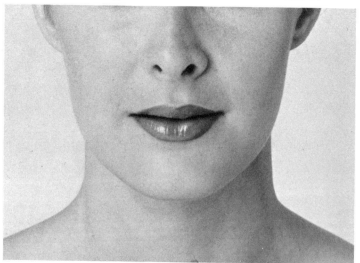

Return head and shoulders to normal position.

Relax while counting 1 and 2 and 3.

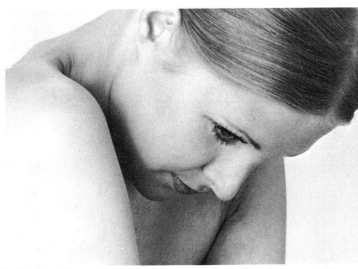

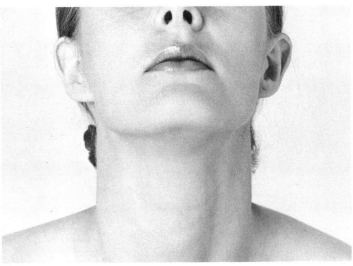

Pull shoulders up as high as possible, chin down and in.
Hold while counting 1 and 2 and 3 and 4 and 5 and 6.

Then slowly stretch head up as you slowly pull shoulders down.
Hold while counting 1 and 2 and 3 and 4 and 5 and 6.

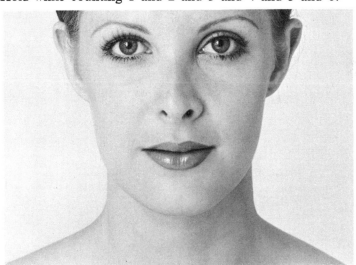

Return to normal position.
Relax while counting 1 and 2 and 3.

Sana-Facial 3
Do 1 Time | NECK

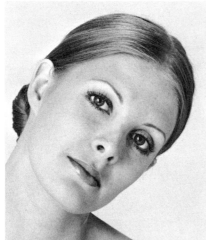 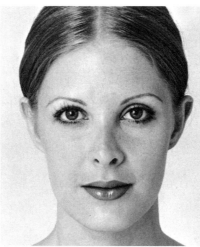 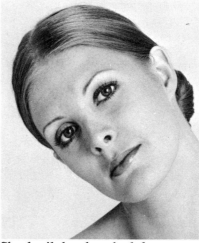 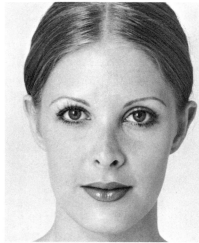

Slowly tilt head to the right.

Hold while counting 1 and 2 and 3 and 4 and 5 and 6.

Return head to normal position.

Relax while counting 1 and 2 and 3.

Slowly tilt head to the left.

Hold while counting 1 and 2 and 3 and 4 and 5 and 6.

Return head to normal position.

Relax while counting 1 and 2 and 3.

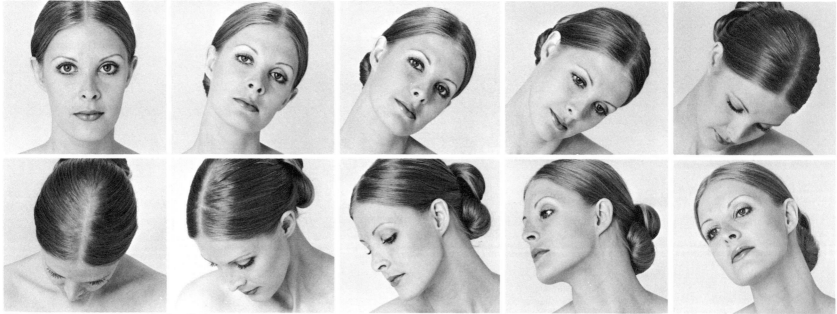

Slowly rotate head in a circle. Only move head. Keep rest of body motionless.

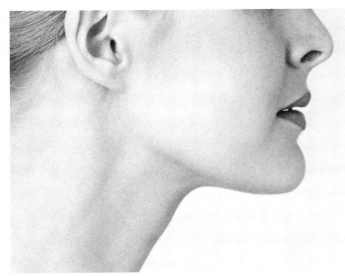

Keep body motionless. Slowly turn head to the right.
Hold while counting 1 and 2 and 3 and 4 and 5 and 6.

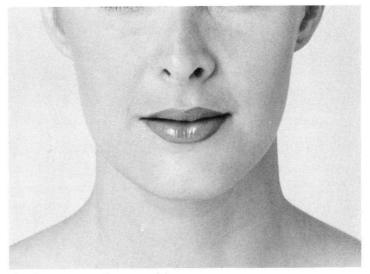

Slowly return to front position.
Relax while counting 1 and 2 and 3.

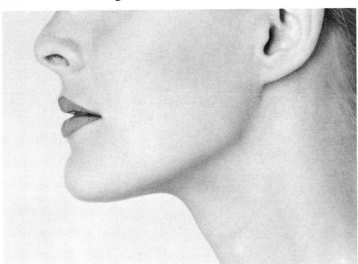

Slowly turn head to the left.
Hold while counting 1 and 2 and 3 and 4 and 5 and 6.

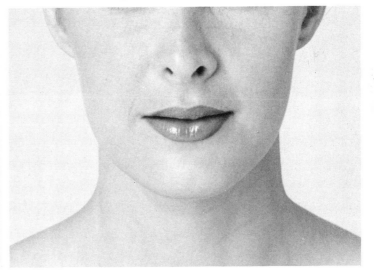

Slowly return to front position.
Relax while counting 1 and 2 and 3.

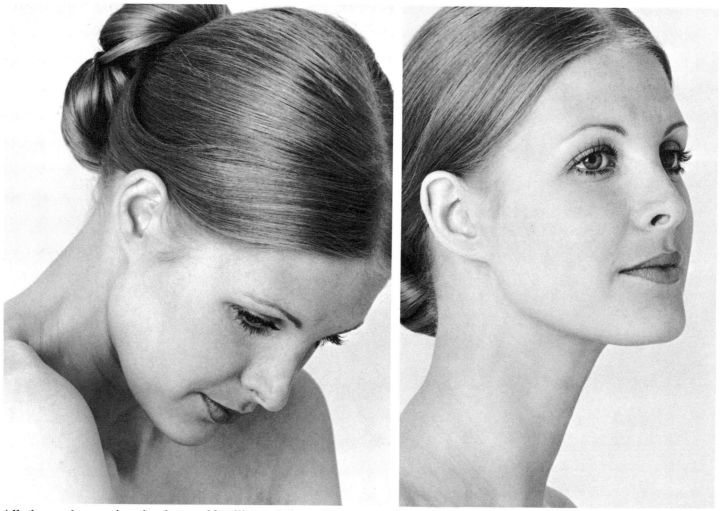

All the neck exercises in the world will not help unless you stretch your neck tall, hold head up, do not slouch.

Sana-Facial 4

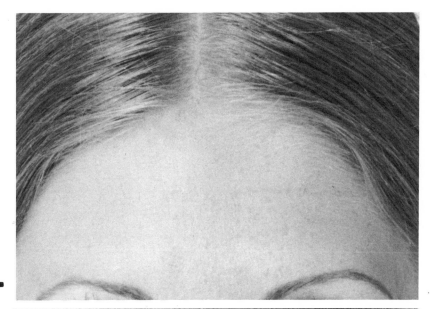

FOREHEAD VERTICAL
AND HORIZONTAL LINES
WRINKLES
SCOWL LINES

Sana-Facial 4
Do 1 Time

FOREHEAD
VERTICAL LINES
LINES NOT DUE TO AGING

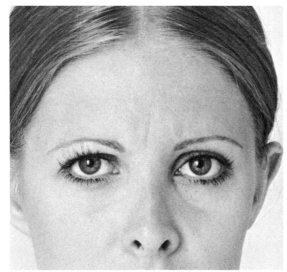

Frown. Notice vertical lines formed.

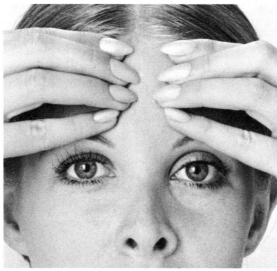

Place 4 fingers behind each vertical forehead line. Stop frowning.

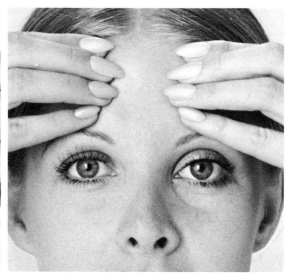

Tightly pull outward while counting 1 and 2 and 3 and 4 and 5 and 6. Stop pulling.

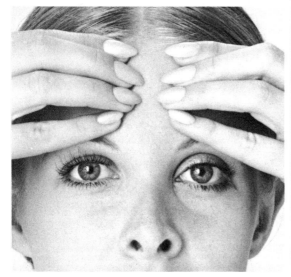

Keep hands on forehead lines.
Relax while counting 1 and 2 and 3.

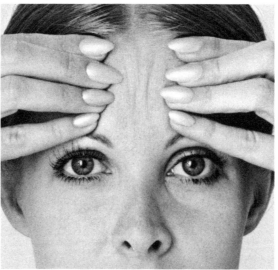

Now push inward while counting 1 and 2 and 3 and 4 and 5 and 6.

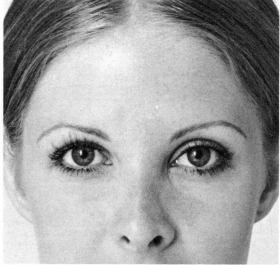

Stop pushing inward. Remove fingers.
Relax while counting 1 and 2 and 3.

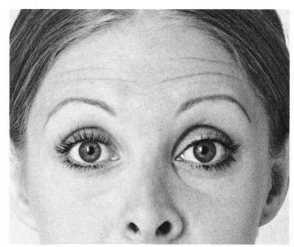

Raise eyebrows as high as you can.

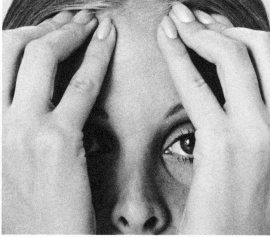

Place 4 fingers of each hand on the top horizontal line on your forehead.

Press tightly against bone.

Push skin upward as far as possible while counting 1 and 2 and 3 and 4 and 5 and 6.

Stop pushing skin upward.

Lower eyebrows to normal.

Hold fingers in place while counting 1 and 2 and 3.

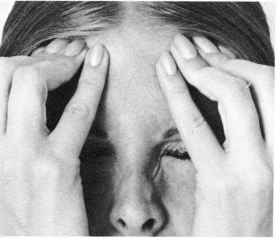

Now move eyebrows downward as far as you can. (Do not scowl — move muscles straight up and down.) Tightly close eyes.

Hold while counting 1 and 2 and 3 and 4 and 5 and 6.

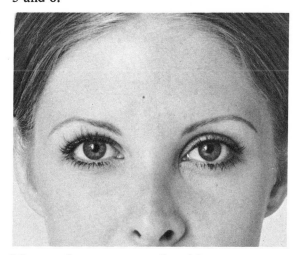

Move eyebrows to normal position.

Open eyes. Remove fingers.

Relax while counting 1 and 2 and 3.

Sana-Facial 4
Do 1 Time

SCOWL LINES

LINES NOT DUE TO AGING

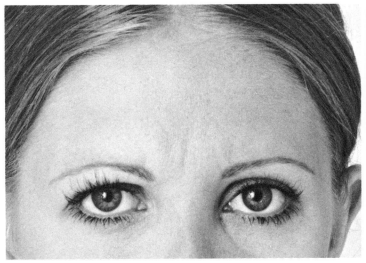

Slowly scowl moving eyebrows together while counting 1 and 2 and 3 and 4 and 5 and 6.

Relax while counting 1 and 2 and 3.

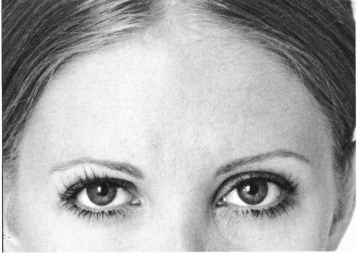

Pull eyebrows in opposite directions as far as possible (use fingers at first if you need help).

Hold while counting 1 and 2 and 3 and 4 and 5 and 6.

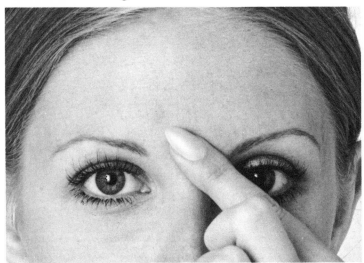

With eyebrows pulled back, place one finger between eyebrows and press in firmly while counting 1 and 2 and 3 and 4 and 5 and 6.

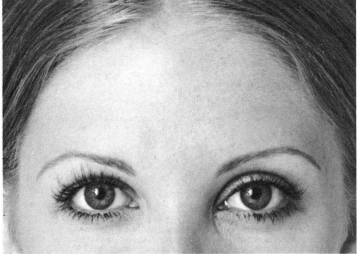

Remove finger.

Relax eyebrows while counting 1 and 2 and 3

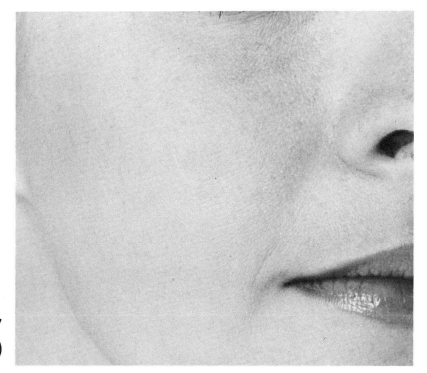

Sana-Facial 5

HOLLOWS BETWEEN NOSE & CHIN

LOWER CHEEKS

UPPER CHEEKS

TEMPLES

POUCHES

JOWLS

Sana-Facial 5

Do 1 Time | CHEEKS

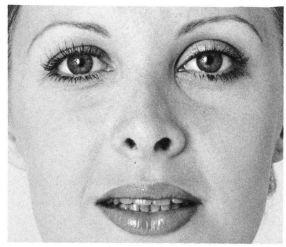

Open mouth.

Keep lips parted and relaxed, teeth together.

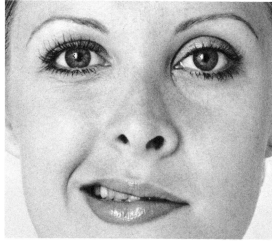

Raise cheek up as shown, on one side, just a little.

(Sneer, but do not push with your lips and do not squint.)

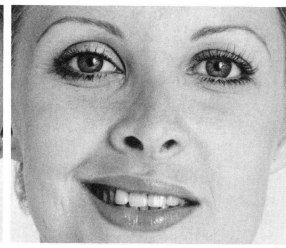

Raise higher.

(Make sure movement is diagonal, *not* horizontal.)

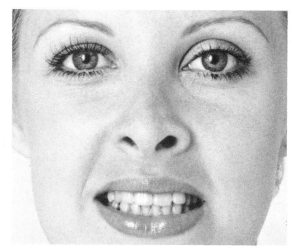

Do both cheeks simultaneously when able.

Hold position while counting 1 and 2 and 3 and 4 and 5 and 6.

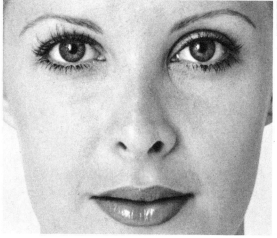

Lower cheek.

Relax while counting 1 and 2 and 3.

Repeat with other side.

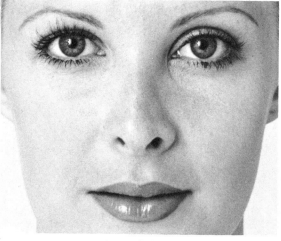

Return to normal closed-mouth position.

Relax while counting 1 and 2 and 3.

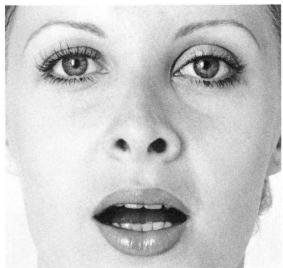

Open mouth.

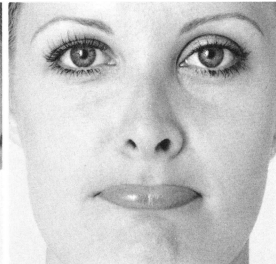

Raise lower teeth and lip over upper lip as far as possible.

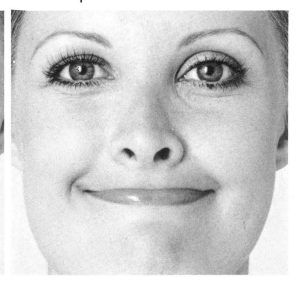

Smile, lifting mouth corners as high as you can.

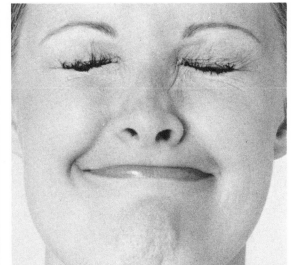

Close eyes tightly.

Hold while counting 1 and 2 and 3 and 4 and 5 and 6.

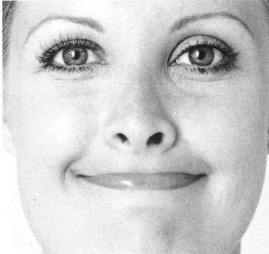

Slowly open eyes.
Lower lip corners.

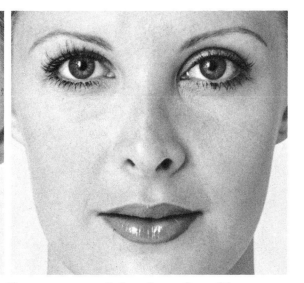

Return to normal closed-mouth position.
Relax while counting 1 and 2 and 3.

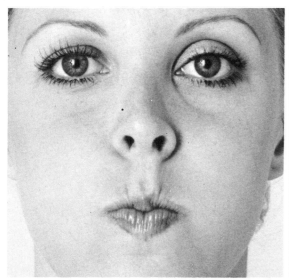

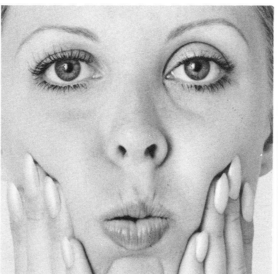

Fill your cheeks with air.

Against this, press in with fingertips allowing air to escape through mouth.

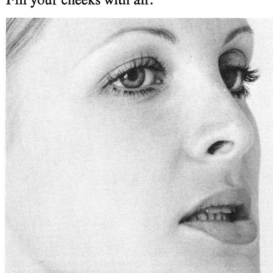

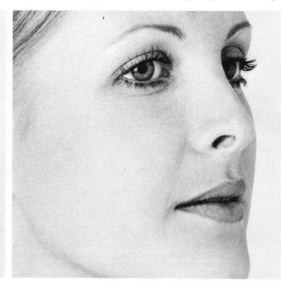

Part lips. Keep teeth closed.
Bite down on back teeth hard. Relax.

Then bite down on back teeth with less pressure.
Relax.

BIBLIOGRAPHY

BIBLIOGRAPHY

Grace Adair, Adairs Cosmetology Examiner (Adair Publ. Co., Miami, Fla., 1937).

Adrienne Ames, Best Face Forward (R. Field, New York, 1947).

Marguerite Agniel, The Art of the Body (Harcourt, Brace & Co., New York, 1931).

The Ancient Art of Beautification (Natural History, New York, Vol. 40).

E. Archer, Let's Face It (Lippincott, Philadelphia, 1959).

Amy Ayer, Facts for Ladies (A.G. Ayer, Chicago, 1890).

H.B. Ayer, Harriet Hubbards Ayer's Book (Home Topics Book Co., New York, 1899).

Dave Aylott, Making the Most of Make-up (London, 1953).

Marguerite Ayriel, The Art of The Body (Harcourt, Brace & Co., New York, 1931).

Beauty (The Butterick Publ. Co., 1890).

Beauty, It's Attainment (The Butterick Publ. Co., 1896).

Polly Bergen, Polly Bergen Book of Beauty (Prentice-Hall, Englewood Cliffs, N.J., 1962).

Louis Paine Benjamin, Why Men Like Us (Stackpole Sons, New York, 1937).

D.G. Brinton, Personal Beauty (W.J. Holland, Springfield, Mass., 1870).

M.A. Burbridge, The Road to Beauty (Greenberg Publ. Inc., New York, 1924).

Margaretta Byers, Designing Women (Simon & Schuster, New York, 1938).

Edith Carter, From Duckling to Swan William-Frederick Press, New York, 1948).

Molly Castle, How to Be 30 For 30 Years (Dodd, Mead, New York, 1962).

Lina Cavalieri, My Secrets of Beauty (Circulation Syndicate, New York, 1914).

Jos. Cherioli, Beauty Culture (Bruce Publ. Co., Milwaukee, 1949).

Jane Clark, The Ladies Guide to Beauty (Garrett & Co., New York).

Dorothy Cochs, Help Yourself To Beauty (Harper & Bros., New York & London, 1935).

Kate Constance, How to Get & Keep A Husband (Dorrance, Philadelphia, 1957).

Florence Courtenay, Physical Beauty (Social Mentor Publications, New York, 1922).

Cozenane, Female Beauty (G.W. Carleton & Co., New York, 1874).

Arnold Jaimes Cozley, The Toilet in Ancient & Modern Times (J.B. Lippincott, Philadelphia, 1873).

E. Crone, Beauty Culture (U.S. Curriculium Laboratory, New Brunswick, N.J., 1962).

John Crum, Beauty & Health (Smith & Darrell, New York, 1941).

John Crum, The Truth About Beauty (Dadd, Mead & Co., New York, 1933).

Bea Danville, Dress Well on $1.00 a Day (W. Funk, New York, 1956).

Gwen Davenport, The Tall Girl's Handbook (Doubleday, Garden City, New York, 1959).

P.M. Armand Day, Famous Beauties in Art (L.C. Page & Co., Boston, 1907).

Veronica Dengel, All About You (Mount Vernon Publ. Co., Mount Vernon, New York, 1953).

E. Duchworth, Visual Beauty Manual (McGraw-Hill, New York, 1950).

Knight Dunlap, Personal Beauty & Racial Betterment (C.V. Mosby Co., St. Louis, 1920).

J. DuPasquier, A Guide To Elegance (Staples Press, London, 1956).

Adelia Ella Fletcher, The Woman Beautiful (Brentano's, New York, 1900).

G. Fran, Art & Craft of Hairdressing (Sir I. Pitman & Sons, Ltd., London, 1936).

Helen Fraser, The Charming Woman (Charming Woman, Inc., New York, 1957).

Fannie Freireich, Applied Science Related to Cosmetology (New York State Vocational And Practical Art Association, Rochester, 1941).

Pauline Furlong, Beauty Culture At Home (Paulette School, Washington, D.C., 1914).

G. Gaines, Secrets of Beauty And Charm (The Concord Press, Lynn, Mass., 1936).

Rita Gam, The Beautiful Woman (Prentice-Hall, Englewood Cliffs, N.J., 1967).

Madge Garland, The Changing Face of Beauty (M. Barrows, New York, 1957).

Gifford, Fundamentals of Beauty (The Hobson Book Press, Cynthiana, Ky., 1944).

Jane Gordon, Home Beauty Treatments (J. Lane, London, 1934).

K. Gray, Lovely To Look At (Link House Publ., London, 1937).

Hairdressing & Beauty Culture (Hairdressers Registeration Council, Sir J. Pitman & Sons, London, 1948).

Hanchel, The Beauty Culture Hanbook (Sir J. Pitman & Sons, Ltd., London, 1935).

"Haper's Bazar Beauty Book," Harpers Bazaar (Appleton-Century, Crofts, New York, 1959).

M. Hart, A Wonderful You (Greenberg, New York, 1947).

Luch Hartzell, How To Visualize Beauty Health (Davis Printing Co., Memphis, 1925).

B.G. Hauser, Mirror, Mirror on the Wall (Farrat, Straus & Cusahy, New York, 1961).

G. Hauser, Eat & Grow Beautiful (Tempo Books, New York, 1936).

Mary Haweis, The Art of Beauty (Chatto & Windres, London, 1878).

Hildegrade, Over 50 – So What! (Doubleday, Garden City, New York, 1963).

John Hope, Art of Feminine Charm (Webjel Publ. Co., Inc., Los Angeles, Ca. 1933).

Edna Hopper, My Secrets of Youth (The Reilly & Lee Co., Chicago, 1925).

Elizabeth Howes, Good Grooming (Little, Brown & Co., Boston, 1942).

Elizabeth Hubbard, Helpful Advice to Women (Pub. by Author, New York, 1910).

Jos. Huddleston, Secrets of Charm (G.P. Putnam's & Sons, New York, 1929).

Terry Hunt, Design for Glamour (Prentice-Hall, New York, 1941).

Isobel (Editor), The Art of Beauty (C.A. Pearson, London, 1899).

"It's Fun To Look & Feel Your Best," Look (New York, 1947).

H. Jameson, The Beauty Box (McLoughlin Bros., Inc., Springfield, Mass., 1931).

Helen Jameson, The Woman Beautiful (Jamieson-Higgins, Co., Chicago, Ill., 1901).

Candy Jones, Finishing Touches (Harper & Rowe, New York 1961).

Ruth Jones, Practical Preparation (Prentice-Hall, Inc., New York, 1939).

Sonya Joslen, The Way To Beauty (Pitman Publ. Corp., New York, 1937).

Annette Kellermann, Physical Beauty (George H. Doran Co., New York, 1918).

C. Kibbee, Standard Textbook of Cosmetology (Milady Publ. Corp., New York, 1951).

J. Lane, Your Carriage Madam (J. Wiley & Sons, Inc. 1947).

E. Lapish, Be Beautiful (D. Appleton & Co., New York, 1932).

Ruth Larison, Those Enduring Young Charms (Harper & Bros., New York, 1942).

LeClaire, LeClaire on Beauty Culture (Mme. LeClaire, Inc., Milwaukee, Wisc. 1937).

Maron Lee, ABC's of Beauty (Lantern Press, New York, 1950).

Lois Leeds, Beauty & Health (J.B. Lippincott, Philadelphia, 1927).

Helen Livingstone, Everyday Beauty Culture (McKnight & McKnight, Bloomington, Ill., 1945).

M.B. Luegen, Professional Cosmetology (Western Printing Corp., Whittier, Ca., 1935).

Alice Long, My Lady Beautiful (Progress Co., Chicago, Ill., 1908).

Renee Long, Style Your Personality (Doubleday, Doram & Co., Inc., New York, 1939).

Mary MacFadyen, Beauty Plus (Emerson Books, Inc., New York, 1938).

L. Malmstead, What Everybody Wants to Know (The Hefferman Press, Spencer, Mass., 1928).

L. Malmstead, Your Face & Figure (The Penn Publ. Co., Philadelphia, 1931).

L. Martin, How To Win A Husband (Bantam Publ., Los Angeles, Ca. 1940).

Elizabeth McGrath, Modern Technique for Beauty Culturists (New Medicine Pub. Co., Chicago, Ill., 1936).

Edyth McLeod, Beauty After 40 (Ziff-Davis, Chicago, Ill., 1949).

Edyth McLeod, How To Sell Cosmetics (The Drug & Cosmetic Industry, New York, 1937).

Edyth McLeod, Lady, Be Lovely (Wilcox & Follett, Chicago, Ill., 1955).

Nora M. McNamara, The History & Trade Analysis of Cosmetology (Western Printing Corp. Whittier, Ca. 1931).

Nora M. McNamara, The Theory & Science of Cosmetology (Adait Publ. Co., Miami, Fla., 1939).

Mary Miller, Here's To You, Miss Teen (Holt, Rinehart & Winston, New York, 1960).

Adena Minott, How To Be Beautiful (Gotham Press, Inc., New York, 1923).

Arthur Moler, Manual of Beauty Culture (Chicago, Ill., 1937).

L. Molmstead, Awaken Your Sleeping Beauty (E.P. Button & Co., Inc., New York, 1935).

Marie Montaigue, How To Be Beautiful (Harper & Bros., New York, 1913).

Lola Montez, The Arts of Beauty (Dick & Fitzgerald, New York, 1858).

Monin, The Hygiene of Beauty (Saberton, Murray & Co., New York, 1893).

Mary Moore, You Can Too (J.J. Tepper Corp., New York, 1950).

Margaret G. Morton, The Arts of Costume & Personal Appearance (J. Wiley & Sons, Inc., 1943).

Anne Murray, Theory of Cosmetology (Anne Murray Publ. Co., Hollywood, Ca. 1942).

Seli Nobel, Glamour & How To Achieve It (Fortuny, New York, 1939).

Mary Phillips, More Than Skin Deep (R.R. Smith, New York, 1948).

John Powers, Secrets of Charm (Winston, Philadelphia, 1954).

Susane Power, The Ugly-Girl Papers (Harper & Bros., New York, 1875).

Frederick H. Radford (Ed.), The Art & Craft of Hairdressing (I. Pitman, London, 1908).

H. Redgrove, Cream of Beauty (W. Heinemann, Ltd., London, 1931).

Miriam Reichl, Person Beauty & Charm Homemakers Encyclopedia (Homemaker's Encyclopedia, New York, 1952).

R. Rockwell, Modren Cosmetology (Prentice-Hall, Inc., New York, 1940).

J. Rohrer, Prof. Rohrer's Handbook on Scientific, etc. (New York, 1911).

Frederick Magee Rossiter, Face Culture, The Value of Your Smile (Pageant Press, New York, 1956).

H. Rubinstein, The Art of Feminine Beauty (H. Leveright, New York, 1930).

H. Rubinstein, Food For Beauty (I. Washburn, New York, 1938).

H. Rubinstein, My Life For Beauty (Simon & Schuster, New York, 1966).

Mildred Ryan, Dress Smartly (Scribner, New York, 1956).

Gertrude Gordon Sachs, My Lady's Handbook (National Library Press, New York, 1938).

E. Sanders, Practical Face Treatment & Natural Beauty (Touslove, Hanson & Combs, Ltd., London, 1902).

Daniel R. Shafer, Secrets of Life Unveiled (Shafer & Co. Ltd., 1877).

C. Shephard, My Lady's Toilette (C.H. Craves, Philadelphia, 1911).

Doree Smedley, You're Only Young Twice (Simon & Schuster , New York, 1941).

Adelaide Smith, Modern Beauty & Barber Science (Prentice-Hall, Inc., New York, 1931).

Joseph H. Smith, The Beauty Specialist's Manual (H.R. Howell Publ. Co., New York, 1930).

Horace Smith, Scientific Fundamentals (H.R. Howell Pub. Co., Brooklyn, N.Y. 1926).

Sozinskey, Personal Appearance (Allen, Lane & Scott, Philadelphia, 1877).

Blanche Staffe, My Lady's Dressing Room (Cassell Publ. Co., New York, 1892).

E. Stanchak, How To Teach Beauty Culture (E.M. Stanchak, Wilkes-Barre, Pa., 1939).

Louis Thomas Stanley, The Beauty of Woman (W.H. Allen, London, 1955).

Margaret Story, How To Dress Well (Funk & Wagnalls Co., New York & London, 1924).

J. Stotter, Beauty Unmasked (The Raymond Press, New York, 1936).

Esmond Szekely, The Golden Door Book of Beauty (Prentice-Hall, Englewood Cliffs, N.J., 1961).

Eve Taylor, Face, Figure, Fashion (Mills & Brown, London, 1968).

D. Teeling, This Side of Your Mirror (Fleet Pub. Corp., New York, 1960).

The Science of Beautistry (The National School of Cosmeticians, Inc., New York, 1932).

Gertrude Thomas, Modern Textbook of Cosmetology (Milady Pub. Corp., New York, 1961).

Albert Turner, The Attainment of Womanly Beauty (The Health-Culture Co., New York, 1960).

Sylvia Ullback, No More Alibis (Photoplay Pubs. Co., Chicago, 1934).

Sylvia Ullback, Pull Yourself Together, Baby! (Macfadden Book Co., New York, 1936).

Helen Valentine, Better Than Beauty (Modern Age Books, Inc., New York, 1938).

Lizalottar Valesca, More Than Beauty (Carlton Press, New York, 1961).

V. Vernon, Beauty Products (Hutchinson & Co., Ltd., London, 1939).

Vogue's Book Of Beauty (The Conde Nast Publications, Inc., 1933).

Emma E. Walker, The Pretty Girl Papers (Little, Brown & Co., Boston, Mass., 1910).

E.E. Walker, Female Beauty (Scofield & Voorhies, New York, 1840).

Alexander Walker, Beauty (H.G. Books, London, 1852).

Alexander Walker, The Book of Beauty (Holland & Glover, New York, 1843).

Mary Young, Charm Is Not Enough (Bookhampton Press, Leicester, 1965).

Florence E. Wall, The Principles & Practice of Beauty Culture (Keystone Publishers, New York, 1941).

Katherine Wellman, Beauty Begins At Home (Covici-Friede, New York, 1936).

C. West, Ageless Youth (Thomas Y. Crowell Co., New York, 1929).

Ernest H. Westmore, Beauty, Glamour & Personality (Prang Co., Sandusky, Ohio, 1947).

P. Westmore, Perfect Make-Up Guide (House of Westmore, Hollywood, Ca. 1934).

Belle Armstrong Whitney, What To Wear (Good Health Publ. Co., Battle Creek, Michigan, 1916).

Kathryn Wilson, The Successful How Dresser (L. Douglas Printing Co., Omaha, Nebr. 1924).

Margery Wilson, You're As Young As You Act (J.B. Lippincott Co., Philadelphia, 1951).

Thomas Wovenoth , Facts & Faces (Published by the Author, London, 1852).

Joyce Wyhes, Cosmetics & Adornment (N.Y. Philosophical Library, 1961).